Dr William Davies graduated in psychology from University College London and completed his postgraduate clinical training at the University of Birmingham, England. He is a Consultant Psychologist and head of APT, The Association for Psychological Therapies, one of the UK's leading providers of training for Mental Health professionals. Dr Davies was previously Head of Psychology at St Andrew's Hospital, Northampton – a national resource for patients needing specialised care. Dr Davies has written and taught numerous courses and workshops, most notably The RAID® Course for working with extreme behaviour, and 'Preventing Face-to-Face Violence', each of which has been attended by well over 10,000 professionals.

The aim of the **Overcoming** series is to enable people with a range of common problems and disorders to take control of their own recovery programme.

Each title, with its specially tailored programme, is devised by a practising clinician using the latest techniques of cognitive behavioural therapy – techniques which have been shown to be highly effective in changing the way patients think about themselves and their problems.

Many books in the Overcoming series are recommended by the UK Department of Health under the Books on Prescription scheme.

Other titles in the series include:

OVERCOMING ANOREXIA NERVOSA
OVERCOMING ANXIETY, 2ND EDITION
OVERCOMING BODY IMAGE PROBLEMS INCLUDING BODY
DYSMORPHIC DISORDER
OVERCOMING BULIMIA NERVOSA AND BINGE-EATING, 2ND EDITION
OVERCOMING CHILDHOOD TRAUMA
OVERCOMING CHRONIC FATIGUE
OVERCOMING CHRONIC PAIN
OVERCOMING COMPULSIVE GAMBLING
OVERCOMING DEPERSONALIZATION AND FEELINGS OF UNREALITY
OVERCOMING DEPRESSION, 3RD EDITION
OVERCOMING DISTRESSING VOICES
OVERCOMING GRIEF
OVERCOMING HEALTH ANXIETY
OVERCOMING HOARDING
OVERCOMING INSOMNIA AND SLEEP PROBLEMS
OVERCOMING LOW SELF-ESTEEM, 2ND EDITION
OVERCOMING MILD TRAUMATIC BRAIN INJURY AND
POST-CONCUSSION SYMPTOMS
OVERCOMING MOOD SWINGS
OVERCOMING OBSESSIVE COMPULSIVE DISORDER
OVERCOMING PANIC AND AGORAPHOBIA
OVERCOMING PARANOID AND SUSPICIOUS THOUGHTS, 2ND EDITION
OVERCOMING PERFECTIONISM
OVERCOMING PROBLEM DRINKING
OVERCOMING RELATIONSHIP PROBLEMS
OVERCOMING SEXUAL PROBLEMS
OVERCOMING SOCIAL ANXIETY AND SHYNESS, 2ND EDITION
OVERCOMING STRESS
OVERCOMING TRAUMATIC STRESS
OVERCOMING WEIGHT PROBLEMS
OVERCOMING WORRY AND GENERALISED ANXIETY DISORDER,
2ND EDITION
OVERCOMING YOUR CHILD'S FEARS AND WORRIES
OVERCOMING YOUR CHILD'S SHYNESS AND SOCIAL ANXIETY
OVERCOMING YOUR SMOKING HABIT

OVERCOMING ANGER AND IRRITABILITY

2nd Edition

A self-help guide using
Cognitive Behavioural Techniques

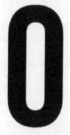

OVERCOMING

WILLIAM DAVIES

ROBINSON

ROBINSON

First published in Great Britain in 2000 by Robinson,
an imprint of Constable & Robinson Ltd
This edition published in 2016 by Robinson

A CIP catalogue record for this book
is available from the British Library.

Important Note
This book is not intended as a substitute for medical advice or treatment.
Any person with a condition requiring medical attention should consult a
qualified medical practitioner or suitable therapist.

ISBN: 978-1-47212-022-9

Typeset in Bembo by Initial Typesetting Services, Edinburgh
Printed and bound in Great Britain by Clays Ltd, St Ives plc

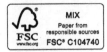

Robinson
An imprint of
Little, Brown Book Group
Carmelite House
50 Victoria Embankment
London EC4Y 0DZ

An Hachette UK Company
www.hachette.co.uk

www.littlebrown.co.uk

To Philippa

Contents

PART THREE

Putting Things Into Practice

Acknowledgements

More of a tribute than an acknowledgement. First to the great names in the therapies on which this book is based: especially B.F. Skinner, A.T. Beck, Albert Ellis, Christine Padesky, and Marsha Linehan. And to another great name, Neil Frude. I co-authored 'Preventing Face-to-Face Violence' with Neil and I am forever indebted to his generosity in our joint work. He is responsible for the 'irritants, costs, transgressions' concept, for much of the central spine of the model that I espouse in this book, and surely for much more. Not only that but he then went on to establish the concept of bibliotherapy and to promote the UK's Books on Prescription scheme, which I am proud to say has adopted this book into its ranks. Also to a great name in anger, Raymond Novaco, for his helpful and interesting observations on the first edition. And to my patients who have given so much of the case material I use, along with their often deliberately entertaining contributions to working on their problems − it seems that people with these problems also have a remarkable sense of humour. And most of all to my wife Philippa who features in a disconcertingly large number of the anecdotes ('Is it me who is irritable or you who is irritating?') and does so cheerfully and apparently without minding. Also for her reading of the book and the invaluable comments she makes in doing so. Finally to Andrew McAleer at Robinson, firstly for prompting this second edition and also for tolerating the ever-shifting 'deadlines' certainly without anger and apparently without irritation. I am grateful to you all.

PART ONE

UNDERSTANDING
WHAT HAPPENS

1

What are anger and irritability?

Anger and irritability belong together because they feed off each other. But they also exist independently, and they also link with other ideas, so I think it is useful to ponder what they are; it helps us tackle something if we know just what it is we are looking at. So let us examine the easier one first, and the easier one is . . . anger.

Anger is particularly interesting because it is often held to be unique amongst the 'negative' emotions in that it has a distinct positive side for some people. This is because, when we are seriously angry, we feel:

1. Very alive
2. Very energised
3. Very right!

What makes it such a dangerous emotion is that it seriously impairs our judgement so, although we may be absolutely convinced we are right in 'the heat of the moment' we find later that we were totally wrong. Moreover, people don't like to see others angry; it makes them feel uneasy and maybe frightened. Certainly it does not lead to a relaxed, positive interaction between people!

As an example of how right people can feel, I have worked with some men in prison who have murdered their wives. And, often enough, at the moment in time at which they did it, it was what they wanted to do, they were convinced they were right to do it. Later on, they cannot believe what they have done or how they could possibly have thought it was the right thing to do and, moreover, they now face a long time behind bars, missing the very person who would have brought them some solace.

You may feel that these men are quite different from you and me, but I am afraid that this is not the case; before the incident in question many of them were unremarkable, just like anybody else. Frequently one hears friends and neighbours say, 'I just can't believe he would do that'.

So, taken to extremes, that is what anger is capable of but, routinely, it can produce results which are very far from what we want or even what we intended. Consider the following account of an incident:

It was a Wednesday evening and four of us went down to town for a meal in an Indian restaurant. That's me, my wife and the two kids. Anyway, we parked the car in a back street, it must have been about eight o'clock in the evening, walked round to the restaurant and had a very good meal. It was the first time we'd been there, we were all on good form, had a good laugh and a joke about

4

everything, even at how thick and new the carpets were, and altogether had a thoroughly good time. Anyway, about half-past nine or ten o'clock, we'd just turned the corner of the street we'd parked the car in when we heard an almighty crash and the sound of breaking glass. Except it hardly sounded like glass, it was a stronger, louder sound than that. We looked down the street, and there was some guy with his head stuck through the passenger window of our car, and another guy standing by him. I didn't grasp what was happening for a moment; then I realised that the sound we had heard was the window glass breaking, and these two were in the process of stealing the radio from my car. Anyway, I felt that mixture of stuff that courses through your body when these things happen, shouted but not very loud, and set off after these two. One guy saw me after a couple of seconds and just ran off. That left the guy with his head still through the window, engrossed in prising the radio out of the car. He still had his head through the window when I got there, I just grabbed hold of him and pulled him out – I didn't care if his head caught on the bits of broken glass or not – and manhandled him, not at all gently, on to the floor. By this time my wife was there and telling me to take it easy, and one of the kids had already got his mobile phone out and was dialling for the police. The lad I'd got out of the car was never more than sixteen, but I just had him on the floor and could cheerfully have throttled him. What did they think they were doing, just thinking they could go up to somebody else's property

5

and take it? Anyway, I just sat astride him, threatening him and telling him what a useless piece of machinery he was until the police came. Half a dozen people must have gone past us during all that, but I couldn't care less. When the police arrived they did at least seem to take my side, took all the details and took him off in their car.

Examples such as this give us a clue as to what happens in the brain when we get angry. The amygdala (a small, almond-sized and almond-shaped part of the brain) is held as responsible for many of our emotions, including anger. In fact, when we get really angry it is sometimes referred to as an amygdala-hijack and this is a powerful and accurate way of thinking of it. Effectively this tiny part of the brain (along with its near neighbours) hijacks the rest of the brain and imposes its will upon it. This is particularly interesting because the amygdala belongs to what is sometimes referred to as our 'primitive brain' in that it is evolutionarily old; it is a part of the brain that all mammals have. So, in effect, what happens is that a primitive part of our brain hijacks the rest of it – the cerebral cortex, the part of the brain that only we have. So, it hijacks our thinking, planning, rational, executive-function part of the brain.

This is well illustrated because you will often hear people say after they have lost their temper 'I don't know what I was thinking of', and this is because they weren't really thinking at all: the thinking part of the brain had been hijacked by the primitive brain. Other colloquial expressions for anger show similar insight. For example you might hear the observation 'he just exploded with rage', and the explosion metaphor is a good one because what is happening in the brain is very much akin to that: the amygdala and the primitive brain in general mount a vicious hijack – by intense neuronal firing – of the rest of the brain before it has time to respond. (The primitive brain always reacts much more quickly than the cerebral cortex, which is why, upon hearing a loud noise, you may duck so quickly that you are virtually moving at the same instant as the noise occurs. This is powered by the primitive brain, so there is no thought behind it, and you may indeed be ducking *into* the imagined missile that you are seeking to avoid. So it is not useful, but it is a good illustration of how the primitive brain reacts so much more quickly than the thinking brain. This phenomenon is put to good effect when we teach people who are under threat from an angry-aggressive assailant to 'play for time', because the longer time goes on the better the chance that the thinking brain will regain control in the angry assailant's mind.)

So, when we 'lose it' this is quite a major event inside our head. It is also very apt phraseology because the 'it' that we are losing is 'control of ourselves'. The control we normally have is through the thinking, executive-function part of the brain (the cerebral cortex) and it is indeed this that we lose when the amygdala hijacks the whole process. And it is not just in the brain, because adrenaline and other substances are pumped through us, our blood vessels change and so on. This is sometimes referred to as the 'fight or flight' response but, in anger, I'm not convinced that this shorthand phrase does it justice: when we 'lose it' we lose a tremendous lot.

I would love to stop there and have us conclude that anger is simply a bad thing and that we must learn to eradicate it. But the fact that you're reading this means that you know better than that, and it does get more complicated. One of the most relevant complications is that the anger stemming from the primitive brain can be harnessed with the cerebral cortex or thinking brain, and this is recognised in the saying 'revenge is a dish best served cold'. What this means is that many people can hang on to their intense anger, then use their 'thinking brain' to plan out how to get even with the person who has angered them.

Michael Winner's 1974 film *Death Wish* gives a graphic description of how this might occur. A break-in occurs during which the hero's (Charles Bronson) wife is raped and mother murdered. Charles Bronson's character subsequently goes on a revenge spree where he lures muggers to attack him and, when they attempt to, shoots them. This was an early example of the revenge-movie genre and I can recollect the sheer delight of the cinema audience each time Charles Bronson shot another 'baddie'.

You might object to this example on the grounds that this is Hollywood, it's not real life, yet, in the forensic world, such revenge crimes are not uncommon. Of course they're neither glossy nor exciting in the way a Hollywood version is, but they can follow the same principle, namely, merging the primitive brain and the cerebral. You might also rightly say that Charles Bronson's character was more than angry – he was bereaved, distraught, devastated, and so on. But this happens often enough in real life; sometimes we experience relatively 'pure' anger, other times it is mixed with emotions such as disappointment, upset, or whatever, but in either case the anger is usually the most powerful driver of what we subsequently do.

Sadly, a similar phenomenon occurs in everyday life, in divorce. A frequent scenario is that one partner tries to keep the marriage together then, their patience eventually snaps and they turn 'angry'. Divorce proceedings begin, lawyers are recruited, and the person's anger – and intellect – are directed towards inflicting the greatest possible suffering and loss on their former partner.

Just to get our terms completely right we have now of course moved into talking about aggression and violence. In this case the aggression and violence is *fuelled* by anger, but, in fact, anger is an emotion and, unless we give vent to it, no one else will necessarily know we are angry. You have probably had a conversation where you have told somebody that you were 'furious' about something and your listener may have expressed surprise – 'I would never have guessed'. And this is the nature of emotions: we can if we wish keep them to ourselves. So, if we are to be pedantic about it, the killing spree that Charles Bronson's character goes on was the *manifestation* of his anger, rather than the anger itself. (The reason this distinction is sometimes made is that we also see aggression and violence in the *absence* of anger. For example, people who rob banks necessarily use aggression or violence – otherwise it would be termed a simple theft

– even though they are probably not angry with the bank employees; in fact they may well never met them before.)

But we are getting away from the point. To summarise: anger is a massive emotion which involves huge things suddenly taking place in our brain and also physically. It is also an emotion which can have life-changing effects for us as a result of the things we do when we are angry. In extreme circumstances it can lead to our incarceration; much more routinely it can lead to the fracturing of our relationships and the damaging of our own happiness.

'Justified' anger: a proportionate response?

One of the main judgements we make when we see someone behaving in an aggressive or hostile way is whether they are *justified* in doing so. If we consider that they are justified, then we probably won't think of that person as having a problem with their anger. After all, everybody gets angry sometimes; we only think of someone having a problem when they are hostile, angry or aggressive *without good cause*. If we think the person is justified in being angry or aggressive, then we tend to see nothing wrong with that. So, if we see David (the guy who was having his radio stolen) as justified in his anger, we probably won't blame him for pinning the thief to the ground until the police arrive. We might see that as a proportionate response. If, on the other hand, he had started banging the sixteen-year-old's head up and down on the pavement while loudly cursing him, we might have seen that as disproportionate and unjustified.

However, sometimes our judgement goes a little hazy. I can still remember the first time I saw the classic film *One Flew Over the Cuckoo's Nest*, in which Louise Fletcher's character Nurse Ratched torments a group of mentally ill patients led by Jack Nicholson's Randall P. McMurphy. Certainly the patients were full of bad feeling towards Nurse Ratched about an hour into the film, but not half as much as the audience. At this point, after Nurse Ratched's particularly savage treatment of one of the patients, McMurphy could stand it no longer, grabbed hold of her, had her on the floor and was throttling the life out of her. Half the audience in the cinema was on its feet, shouting encouragement and hoping he would finish the job before the two male nurses rushing to Ms Ratched's assistance could get there. He didn't, the authorities got the better of him, and we all later trudged unhappily out of the cinema.

Even though Nurse Ratched's behaviour was extreme, perhaps McMurphy's response was somewhat disproportionate. Of course, in a case like this our judgement is clouded by the events being on the silver screen rather than taking place in reality. But this 'temporary clouding of judgement' is exactly the problem; because, unfortunately, it happens not just on the silver screen but in real life as well. On those occasions we get repeatedly remorseful and self-critical. We say we 'overreacted' or 'don't know what got hold of us'. We feel that our response was out of all proportion to the event; it was not *justified*.

These are themes that will run throughout this book. How do we get ourselves to respond to negative events in a way that is *in proportion* to them? In a way that we, and others, would say is *justified*?

We sometimes like to see people getting angry, so long as they are on our side. Margaret Thatcher was often referred to as 'handbagging' her counterparts from other European countries in order to stick up for what many in Britain perceived as their rights and few people complained about that at the time. (Her contemporary, Ronald Reagan, did something similar on the other side of the Atlantic, but in a more charming way.) Margaret Thatcher's successor John Major, on the other hand, was painted as a much greyer character (literally in the case of the satirical *Spitting Image* programme): so grey, in fact, that he would be unlikely to get openly angry with anyone. Whether this perception was accurate is another matter but, accurate or not, it seemed to count against him. What is more, this negative perception of John Major was exacerbated by rumours that he could also be irritable in private – a shade on the snappish side when perhaps it wasn't warranted. Again, whether this perception was true is another matter, but it does illustrate the point that what people dislike is not the fact of other people getting angry, it's the fact of other people reacting in a way that is not justified, or out of proportion to the situation.

One final but important thought: how are we to judge what is reasonable and proportionate? We have already seen that what seems perfectly reasonable 'in the heat of the moment' seems like a tragic overreaction later on. So what is our yardstick? Here are a couple of ideas.

For me, I like to think of a wise old judge listening quietly to me describing exactly what happened and then coming to a judgement. For example, with David, he might say, 'Yes, I think if I were a younger man and I came across somebody breaking into my car I too would want to pull him out of it and sit on him until the police arrived. I think that is a reasonable and proportionate response.' I find this a very good yardstick.

A lot of people use Facebook in a similar way. In other words, they describe an event and their reaction to it and then see what their Facebook friends think of it. As a yardstick for judging how proportionate a response is I think this has some promise. In fact, so long as we give an impartial account of what happened and what our response was, and so long as our friends are a reasonable representation of society, then this can be excellent. In fact, we don't even have to use Facebook; we can simply *imagine* what the general Facebook reaction would be if we were to describe an event and our reaction to it. We can make an internal judgement as to whether what we did – or are thinking of doing – is reasonable and proportionate.

Irritability

Irritability is possibly even more interesting than anger. Several years ago, when the wonderful publishers of this book were urging me to write it, they told me that 'irritability is the second most common problem that people go to their physicians with'. That was the clincher for me

13

and, even though I have no idea where they got that 'statistic' from, I instantly agreed to write it, pausing only to ask 'What was number one?' (Apparently it is 'Doctor, I feel tired all the time', which is so common, I am assured, that physicians simply abbreviate it to TATT.)

I also felt that the good people at Robinson must have sensed that I was a natural-born expert on irritability. After all, when young, my mother would frequently tell me how irritating I was, and I strongly suspect she had a point. So I early on mastered being irritating, but I also knew about the other side if it – being irritable. I can distinctly remember being fifteen years old and sitting round the family dinner table thinking how sad it was that I could never get married because I was so irritable that there couldn't possibly be a girl anywhere in the world that I could tolerate for a whole lifetime.

So, to me, irritability, irritation, irritating, are all ordinary English words that need no explanation whatsoever; I was brought up both irritating and irritable. But it seems this is not universally the case. For example, I have written a three-day course – based on this book – for my fellow professionals and, when it was having one of its inaugural runnings, the guy who was tutoring it phoned me up after half a day to say, 'They want to know what irritability is'. My instant reaction was to reflect that the questioner himself is a consultant clinical and forensic psychologist and surely knew what irritability was. My second reaction was that, if *he* didn't know clearly enough what it is, then probably there are a lot of people who don't.

So, what is irritability? A clever colleague of mine told me that irritability, unlike anger, is 'a predisposition rather than an emotion'. But, while this may be true, I'm not convinced that it totally sums up the nature of irritability. So let's change the word slightly, and ask what it means if we describe somebody as irritable. Perhaps someone who is irritable is someone who becomes angry too easily. That is part of it, although I think we would more likely describe such a person as 'bad-tempered' rather than irritable. 'Irritable' seems too lightweight a word to describe someone who gets angry too easily. Closer might be when we use irritable to describe someone who gets annoyed too easily. So maybe 'annoyable' might be a good synonym for irritable, if only that word existed.

In fact I looked up synonyms of irritability and this is what I found: tetchiness, testiness, touchiness, scratchiness, grumpiness, moodiness, grouchiness, crotchetiness, cantankerousness, curmudgeonliness, churlishness, peevishness, crossness, pique, impatience, fractiousness, crabbiness, waspishness, prickliness, crustiness, shrewishness. They are all good, aren't they, but I still think that to say that someone who is irritable is someone who gets annoyed easily, pretty much sums it up.

And what can we be irritated with? The answer of course is that, if we are irritable, we can be irritated with lots of things. For example, in the UK, even in times of austerity, it seems we still have enough money that we can deliberately build bumps onto perfectly good roads. Apparently we haven't got enough money to fill in the potholes, but we have got plenty to build bumps. (Just in case you are reading this in a country that is sensible enough not to build bumps onto its roads, in the UK we have this system of slowing traffic down by building bumps that jar the car when you go over them, so you have to drive slowly. 'Doesn't that damage the car's suspension, the steering, and the tyres?' you may ask, to which the answer is of course, 'Yes'.)

But there are smaller things as well, aren't there? I like a nice shirt so, the last time we were in Venice, having saved up for fifty years or so, I decided I could buy myself a nice Italian shirt. So I went into one of the many smart shirt shops, chose one I liked the look of and handed over my Euros. Just walking out of the shop I turned back to the assistant and asked her whether my shirt had been made in Italy (I had noticed that some shops had notices in them saying 'All our shirts are made in Italy'). 'No,' she replied, 'it is an Italian fabric but the shirt is made in another country' (then named it).

That's fine, I thought, and said, 'That is a perfectly fine country too' (I'm avoiding saying which country because one of the things that delights me is that this book is purchased in many different languages, and I don't want to alienate an entire nation). So I got my shirt home and tried it on and sure enough it was a fine shirt made of a nice fabric, a good fit, and it looked okay even with me in it. So all was well? No, not quite, because the buttonholes were only just big enough to get the buttons through. Fastening each button involves a tussle and a struggle. I bought the shirt a year ago and it is still a fight to get into it. So this irritates me. It slightly annoys me. It contrasts with other shirts I have which are the exact opposite: they have vertical button holes through which the buttons go easily and, as the icing on the cake, the last buttonhole is horizontal so you automatically know when you have finished your buttoning task. This always has the opposite effect of irritating me – it always slightly pleases me that shirt-makers can be so thoughtful and so meticulous.

As you read this, you must be thinking, 'For goodness sake there are more important things to worry about than the exact size of the buttonholes in your shirt' and you are of course right. Even as I write it, I think exactly the same thing. But this is one of the characteristics about 'irritations' that gives them their power: not only are they irritating but, to rub salt into our wounds, we feel we are making a fuss about nothing. We feel bad and yet we know that no one is about to make us feel better – not even ourselves. Furthermore, there are so many irritations that they can completely ruin the quality of our lives. After all, if one can be irritated about the size of button holes, there is nothing that is safe.

Irritation is also a paradoxical feeling. For example, I recently read a biography of P.G. Wodehouse in which the author said of him that 'He led a long and enjoyable life because he learned early on that nothing really matters'. At first sight that seems idyllic – he would never get irritated or worried, then – but on second sight would we really want to live a life where nothing seems to matter? Of course the thing about irritability is that small things can appear to matter too much. But surely that is better than having them matter not at all? And yet having things matter too much also leads to distress, and therein lies the conundrum: if things matter too much there's a problem, if things don't matter enough there is a problem. Getting it just right is the problem we have to solve.

If you are an unusually kind person you may be thinking, as you read this, 'No, this is all perfectly reasonable, I get really irritated with bumps on the road, and I would be really irritated if the buttonholes on my shirt – or blouse – were too small.' If so, that is wonderful, but I have to tell you that things are about to get worse . . .

It is possible to be irritated about absolutely nothing. I can assure you this is true, because I have first-hand experience of it; it is perfectly possible to wake up feeling irritable. Not actually irritated with anyone or anything, simply aware that you are feeling irritable at the moment. Knowing that if the slightest potentially irritating thing happens, you will become *really* irritated. It is different from feeling depressed or feeling worried; it's a very distinct feeling all of its own. Perhaps depression and anxiety can cause people to be irritable, but they're not the same as it, and people who are neither depressed nor anxious – as well as those who are – can easily be irritable and angry. Anger and irritability can be caused by all sorts of things which we will examine in the rest of this book.

Finally for now, one of the great things about writing this book is the feeling of validation I get in doing so. I know that for you to be reading it – either because it is especially relevant to you, or to a friend or relative, or to a patient – you have recognised the power of irritation and irritability as well as the more widely recognised power of anger. I do hope it lives up to your expectations. By way of reassurance, in spite of my concern at the age of fifteen, I have managed (or maybe my wife has) more than forty years of marriage, so it just shows – these problems can be solved!

Summary

- Irritability and anger take lots of different forms. Both are emotions that most people have felt.
- There's nothing wrong with being angry in itself; sometimes it is clearly justified. It is when we overreact, responding in a way that is out of proportion to the situation, that we lay ourselves open to criticism. And sometimes we ourselves are our harshest critics.
- The very term 'irritability' implies that the reaction is unjustified. It normally suggests that a person is being snappy and bad-tempered when there is no call to be so. As such it fails the 'Justified?' test; people are almost always criticised for being irritable. Again, we may be our harshest critics in this respect.
- There are times when, through frustration or for other reasons, we lose our sense of perspective.

> It's on those occasions that we find ourselves unable to judge what is justified. And then we see ourselves doing things which we feel are justified at the time but which later on – once our true sense of judgement returns – we are horrified that we did.

A final thought

Most of us feel rather critical of irritable and unjustifiably angry people, almost as if they were doing it deliberately to make our lives miserable. And, certainly, it is no fun at all living with an irritable and unjustifiably angry person.

One point that is sometimes forgotten, however, is that neither is it any fun *being* the irritable and angry person! Many, many people have their lives virtually ruined by their own irritability and anger. So it is *both* for them *and* for those around them that this book is written.

Optional exercises

A: Either write or make a mental note of your answers to the following:

1. Are you mainly concerned about your anger, your irritability, or both?

2. Why are you concerned about it or them?
3. What do you put your anger or irritability issues down to?
4. At this early stage of reading the book, what do you think might help you with your anger or irritability?

B: Search YouTube and view these interviews where things don't go according to plan:

1. Clive Anderson interviewing the Bee Gees
2. Russell Harty interviewing Grace Jones
3. Michael Parkinson interviewing Rod Hull and Emu

Do you agree with me that the Bee Gees' anger was justified and proportionate and that Grace Jones's was not? (It doesn't matter if we don't agree – we all have our own views and it's important that we do.) What about Rod Hull using Emu to attack Michael Parkinson? I think that was aggression without anger – what do you think?

2

Hostility, aggression and violence

These are three more words we need to look at. Let's examine hostility first. There is plenty of evidence that we human beings are simply hostile to one another, whether we are angry or not. It is estimated that the United States spends $1.5 trillion on 'defence' annually. So if you can imagine $1000 and then 1000 times that, and then 1000 times that, and then 1000 times that, and then add on half as much again, that is what the United States spends every year. It would be great to think that's this is just a quirk of the United States, but I'm afraid it's not; search online to find the top 100 countries in terms of expenditure.

So where does all this money go? It goes largely on research, development and production of armaments. And these activities are not being done by angry people; these are people who get up in the morning and commute to work, have meetings about what could be done to improve the effectiveness of the drones they are working on, or the next model Kalashnikovs they are developing, or the barrel bombs they are thinking of pushing out of aircraft, or whatever. Then maybe have a cup of coffee, and then get to work improving the lethality of whatever it is they are working on. So these people are not acting whilst in a fit of rage, later to regret a reckless action; they are working for a salary, working at something they may well enjoy doing and be particularly good at – indeed they will have been chosen because they are particularly good at it. This seems to me to be a particularly hostile kind of activity.

You may well say, as plenty of people do, that this is not at all a hostile activity, but a necessary precaution against the hostility of others. What this means then is that all the countries in the world are spending a lot of money on armaments, to protect against the hostility of others. That means, whichever way you look at it, there seems to be agreement that, worldwide, there is a great deal of hostility.

Once you start looking for it, hostility is everywhere. I have just been interrupted by an assistant and, having dealt with the task in hand, we exchanged a few words about the soccer match yesterday. Twenty minutes from the end our team was losing 2–0. By the end of the game our team had won 3–2. I said to my assistant, 'Did you hear what the opposing manager said last night; he said that he had never felt worse in his entire life?' What do you think my assistant's reaction was? Did she say, 'Oh that's a shame, but still I'm glad we won'? Did she say, 'Oh no, that's completely spoilt it for me'? Or did she simply fall around laughing? You've probably guessed right.

Of course we begin making excuses for this too. We can say, 'No, surely he didn't really feel worse than he had ever done in his life' or we can say, 'Yes, but it's only a game, this isn't really hostility, it's just what you do when you're talking about soccer' and so on. In fact, each time we see hostility in ourselves and others, it's easy to make a rationalisation of it; we become really good at doing so. (Later on, I will argue that we don't do ourselves a favour by doing this; I think it's usually best if we are open with ourselves about our emotions and then look at how to handle them.)

Another example. My wife and I were in London recently, walking back to the station after an evening out. It was dark by then, and we reached a point where we could go along either of two streets: one was nicely lit, the other wasn't. Naturally (I would say) we chose the well-lit street. Was this through fear that if we went along the darkened street, we would bump into over-friendly people who would want to talk to us and therefore result in us missing our train? No, it was because we might bump into somebody who wanted to attack us or rob us. Which all goes to show that I must be a particularly paranoid person? No, I don't think so. I think that most people would have chosen to go down the well-lit street, for exactly the same reason as we did.

One last example: schadenfreude. As I'm sure you know, schadenfreude is 'taking pleasure in the misfortunes of others'. Quite a hostile thing to do, wouldn't you say? I think so too, and yet it is very widespread; I cannot ever remember having to explain to anybody why the misfortunes of others should be pleasurable, or anybody ever expressing amazement that people find others' misfortunes pleasurable in any way. Indeed, lots of very fine comedies are based on watching people tripping up, falling over, and otherwise coming to grief. Indeed, all the 'candid camera' home-movie based TV programmes hinge on exactly this. And of course, the icing on the cake is that, in English, we retain the German word for it, just as a hostile little dig at the Germans. (Yes, I'm afraid to tell you if you are reading this in German, that this is what happens; we invent lots of new words every year but we have always been happy to retain schadenfreude, as though this quirk of human nature was unique to German-speakers. But, be assured, it is not.)

So, let's accept that I have made the case that there is plenty of hostility in the world. You could equally make the case that there is plenty of kindness in the world. Most people are distressed if one of their family is distressed. People will risk their lives – and sometimes therefore lose their lives – in an attempt to help others. People will give up one of their own healthy kidneys so that somebody they have never met can benefit from it, and not even allow the stranger to know of their identity; such is their unselfishness that they don't even seek gratitude. I have sometimes collected for charity outside a big supermarket and, often enough, people will come out of the supermarket laden with shopping and perfectly entitled to 'not notice' me standing there. But, again often enough, they will deliberately come over to me, put down all their many bags of shopping, find their handbag (usually it is a woman) and pull out sometimes significant amounts of money. They are never going to see me again, but still they do it.

So what are we to make of this? Is it that there are plenty of hostile people about but there are also plenty of nice people about? I don't think so; I think they are one and the same people. Speaking personally, I have done things I'm ashamed of and I have had thoughts I would be ashamed of if anybody else knew about them; equally, though, I have done things I would love to tell you about and have spent lots of time thinking about how I can help people. And I suspect I am typical, I suspect that just about everybody is capable of hostility and also capable of great kindness. In fact, most people have such a variety of different roles to fulfil, such a range of competing pressures on them, that it is amazing that we are able to balance these things at all. To me it is no wonder that often enough we 'explode' and the whole system collapses; to me the wonder is that, for the most part, we are able to 'keep it together'.

Which brings us on to why I think it is a good idea to admit to our hostility, if and when it occurs. I believe it works best, if we feel hostile for no particularly good reason, simply to accept that fact. The danger is that we find ourselves feeling hostile to somebody and take from that that we must be angry with them. Furthermore, they must therefore have done something to anger us. So now we're not only feeling hostile, we are also angry, also blaming the other person for having done something bad. This kind of thinking can spiral out of control very rapidly. Much better just to accept – if we can – that it is sometimes part of the human condition; that sometimes it is just how life is.

Hostility, like anger, is something we can keep to ourselves if we want to. Nobody need know we are feeling angry or hostile unless we choose to tell them, or unless we give it away by what is termed 'non-verbal leakage', or unless we act in an angry or hostile way. And the term 'hostility' is most often used in relation to acts rather than thoughts and feelings, much like the term 'aggression', which is almost entirely used for acts, and is the term we need to look at next.

So other people may or may not know when we are angry, they even may or may not know when we feel hostile, but they certainly know when we are aggressive. That is the whole point of aggression. And aggression can come in many forms. It includes violence, where one person assaults another either directly or by using a weapon, but it also includes verbal means where one person can shout at, insult, berate or otherwise harass somebody else. That's not the limit of it though; 'sulking' is, typically, an aggressive act and it can be a very powerful one for people who perceive themselves to be in a less powerful position, children for instance. Its power lies in the fact of it being very difficult for the target of the sulking to do anything about, the sulker isn't 'doing anything', after all. So it is a very effective aggressive act and one which some people get attached to throughout their lives. (What happens is that the act of sulking is associated with good feelings – feelings of power and effectiveness – right in the most primitive parts of the brain. This means that we can become attached to sulking irrationally, because the deepest part of the brain is not the rational part. One of my patients reported that she could go into a sulk 'for no reason at all' and described how she arrived at work one day and suddenly found herself in a sulk lasting several hours, for absolutely no reason. Someone I know very well, Sami, says how his father could sulk for three days, and in fact that was the typical length of his sulking period; his mother described it as 'being in a mood'.)

Another hostile or aggressive act involves destroying the property of others. This is much loved by the popular newspapers who seem to relish each time the deserted girlfriend or wife gets her own back on her former lover by chopping all the legs and arms off his favourite suits, battering his Lamborghini, or otherwise mutilating his favourite property. Most people, living in less affluent circumstances, of course find equivalents which are just as satisfying but less often hit the headlines.

The final hostile act, or act of aggression, I want to look at is talking maliciously about other people. Until recently we could do this behind people's backs and this still works in just the same way; malicious gossip behind the other person's back is clearly a hostile or aggressive act which is quite difficult for the victim to respond to. Even if he confronts the gossip, it is usually denied. The digital age has provided an additional channel for this kind of activity. It is easy to text or email people with gossip about a mutual acquaintance, but this is just a digital equivalent of what has happened for centuries. The additional aspect occurs through 'reviews' and through social sites such as Facebook. TripAdvisor-type review sites have given people a new sense of power which some people use really well and, as ever with power, some people seem keen to misuse. The relative anonymity may invite that whereas you might fear retribution if you complained in person.

There is one outstanding arena, however, where this fear of retribution doesn't seem to hold any power. I have a mother-and-son patient combination at the moment, where the thirteen-year-old son is being given an absolutely terrible time by his 'friends' at school, including via Facebook. His parents know about it but feel powerless to act; they feel that if they did then it would be all the worse for their son, and that even if they approached the miscreants' parents about it, this too would get back to their son in some bad way. And they are not alone; this is a frighteningly widespread problem. My friend and colleague Paul Gaffney estimates that around a thousand children a year don't make it from junior school to middle school in Ireland where he lives. Ireland has a population of around five million, so we can calculate that out for other countries. (As far as I know it is not a problem specific to Ireland.) Although this is clearly a very hostile and aggressive act, it is not fuelled by anger, there is no suggestion that my patient's 'friends' are angry with him, and this seems to be the normal way of things in these atrocious bullying incidents.

Aggressive but not angry

When we are angry we may well say and do hostile and aggressive things but, although this may be a very bad idea for us, it is in a way understandable. But what about people who are hostile and aggressive without being angry, why could that be?

The first answer is that there is something in it for the person concerned. For example, a bank robber may well be hostile and aggressive (in fact, as I've already said, he has to be, otherwise it's not classed as robbery), but he has usually not met the bank staff before, so is presumably not angry with them. The hostility and aggression is simply a means to an end, simply a way of getting the staff to hand over the money.

At a slightly different level, we may be hostile and aggressive when we go back to a shop demanding a refund for some faulty goods. Normally we wouldn't be of course; we would simply go back and ask for a refund. But supposing that refund is not forthcoming, then what do we do? The answer depends on who we are of course; some of us will walk off disappointed, but others of us will resort to hostility and aggression to see whether that will give better results. This is often referred to as 'getting angry with them', but whether there is any anger involved is an open question. Certainly there is hostility and aggression, but is it synthesised to gain a good result, or is it really fuelled by anger?

The same thing applies in the domestic situation. Parents will often recount how they 'had to get angry with' their son or daughter before he or she would tidy the bedroom. And yet the very phraseology, that they 'had to' get angry gives away the fact that this was something that was well under control and being used to gain the desired end rather than for any reason otherwise.

Sometimes a distinction is made between 'angry aggression' (hostility and aggression that is fuelled by anger) and 'instrumental aggression' (hostility and aggression that is instrumental in gaining what the person wants). As far as this book is concerned, the clue is in the title; we will be focusing mainly on anger and irritability and things that stem from those. Not exclusively though, because the subjects of aggression, hostility and violence are so important and interact so much with anger and irritability that it is less than useful to confine ourselves too much. In any event, most people have a mixture of motivations for their aggression or hostility: sometimes anger, sometimes some other reason.

Violence

Violence is, in a way, much more straightforward. Everybody knows what violence is; it is damaging physical contact – either without or with a weapon – from one person to another. Sometimes people refer to 'verbal violence' to make the point that words can be very destructive, but I think that is unnecessary and confusing; most of us are perfectly willing to accept that words can be very destructive without invoking the idea of verbal violence.

There is an obvious point about violence that it is probably worth making now even so: violence is dangerous. People can and do lose their lives or suffer life-changing injuries as a result of violence. It is also important to note that the person who gets most damaged is sometimes the person who initiates the violence. For example, David, who went and grabbed hold of the guy who was stealing the radio from his car, may well have been putting himself in a very great deal of danger. In the event, it didn't work out like that, but he was in such a 'blind rage' that he made no assessment of the risk involved. Had the thief been more physically adept, the victim of the theft could well have lost his life or been very badly injured. And this routinely happens, so we need to bear it in mind constantly.

Summary

- Sometimes we can feel hostile for no good reason, and maybe it's best if we recognise this rather than thinking that somebody must have done something to make us angry.
- Aggression is different from anger and irritability. People always know if we are aggressive. There are lots of forms of aggression including physical violence but also hostile words and acts, and 'passive-aggression' usually referred to as sulking.
- Violence is one form of aggression and involves one person assaulting another either with or without a weapon. For us to get involved in violence is dangerous; violence is a very high-risk activity.

Optional exercises

Near the beginning of the chapter I talked about how it is no wonder that we sometimes 'lose it'; the real wonder is how we manage to keep things together for so much of the time. Paul Gilbert writes very well about this in his books on compassion-focused therapy. (The idea here is that one learns to be compassionate to oneself, to understand all the different pressures that assail us.) Where relevant, I incorporate some of Paul's ideas into this book, but you may wish to read them first-hand, in which case I suggest you search online for 'Paul Gilbert compassion focused therapy'.

Some questions you may like to answer:

1. Do you find that you sometimes feel hostile for no good reason, i.e. when you're not angry?
2. If you do sometimes feel hostile for no good reason, have you ever in the past assumed that somebody must have made you feel like this?
3. If you do sometimes feel hostile for no good reason, do you think you could simply accept that fact?
4. Are you ever aggressive to other people? If so what form does your aggression most often take?
5. If you are sometimes aggressive to others, what is the biggest reason you would like to cut it out?
6. Do you ever get involved in violence? If so, have you previously recognised the risk you put yourself at, either in terms of physical harm or in terms of fracturing important relationships or in terms of arrest?

3

What makes us angry?

It is important to know just what makes you angry, because when you come to doing something about it this will be a very important starting point. Clearly, if you know what things make you angry, you can either avoid those things (if possible!) or work out how you would prefer to respond when they happen.

So what kind of things are we looking for? It is said that we are all different, but in fact there tend to be certain themes which produce anger in most people. And remember, we said in Chapter 1 that there is nothing wrong with anger in itself, so long as it is in proportion to the event. What makes us feel bad is when we act out of proportion to what is happening: when we are 'snappy' in the face of no reasonable provocation, or angry in response to something that would normally just mildly irritate most people, or completely 'lose our cool' in response to something that most people would just get irritated or annoyed about.

Irritants, costs and transgressions

So what makes most of us angry? My colleague Neil Frude,

with whom I wrote 'Preventing Face-to-Face Violence', high-lights three main categories: irritants, costs and transgressions.

Irritants

The number of *irritants* in life is boundless. I was talking recently to Aisha, who said she could no longer stand the way her husband ate. Simply the noise his mouth made in chewing his food drove her crazy. Moreover, as so often happens, now she had noticed this, she was waiting for it every mealtime; and that made it ten times worse. It had become a symbol for all that was wrong with him (self-centred, greedy) and with their marriage (she saw him as a different type of person from herself).

People sniffing, coughing, blowing their noses can also be irritating. This certainly used to be the case for me. I sometimes run training events where I spend three days with perhaps a dozen people. Occasionally one of that dozen will have a chronic, hacking cough which lasts for the duration of these three days and longer, for all I know. Certainly I used to find that very irritating indeed. A cough can be so loud; and sometimes its owner seemed deliberately to cough just as I was coming out with an extremely good point! So then I'd have to repeat it and the effect was spoilt. (I cured myself of this sensitivity when I realised that, very often, the owner of the cough would have been perfectly entitled to stay at home, off sick, for the three days. I was therefore able to reinterpret his coughing presence as a compliment to myself: evidence that he simply could not bear to miss out on the event. Whether this is actually true or not doesn't really matter to me; I feel it is true – or at least it could be true – and that keeps me satisfied.)

Neighbours are another excellent source of irritation. Apartments and town houses give everybody great scope for irritating each other. When we were first married, my wife and I lived in a house where we could even hear the neighbours turning on and off their electric switches at the wall sockets, as clearly as if they were in the room with us. That in itself hardly counts as an irritant, but there is plenty of potential for serious irritation: loud music, raised voices, banging picture-hooks into walls, do-it-yourself activity, playing ball games in the street (and on *your* garden) and so on and so on. Not infrequently people's lives are made a complete misery by the sheer level of irritation provoked by their neighbours.

Costs

The cost to you of somebody else's behaviour may be a literal, financial cost, or it may be a cost in terms of time, or in terms of loss of 'face', or indeed any other loss. The common thread here is that, by virtue of what they do, someone costs you in some way; and that makes you angry. Examples include parents being angry when their children break things (because of the financial cost of replacing them); or your spouse being angry because you have crashed the car (again because of the cost of repairing it, or the increased insurance premiums that result).

Interestingly, these kinds of causes of anger sometimes illustrate a 'hangover' effect. Lola told me how angry she was that her thirteen-year-old son had broken a mug by dropping it on the kitchen floor accidentally. When I asked her exactly why it was that she had become angry she said, 'Well, it's the cost of replacing these things; he goes around as though money grows on trees, thinks that whatever he breaks will just automatically get replaced.' I found this strange, because Lola was very far from being poor, and was well able to replace a broken mug or two. But she had not always been wealthy; at one time in her life it would have made a significant impact on her finances to have to buy a new mug, and that frame of mind had stayed with her. Old habits die hard. And there is another possible explanation, too, which you may have spotted; but we will come to that later.

Nicole was telling me how she had taken her five-year-old daughter to a hospital outpatient clinic. She got there promptly for her 2 p.m. appointment but was not seen until approximately two hours later, 4 p.m. What especially enraged her was that she realised after a while that every single person in the clinic had been given an appointment for 2 p.m., and the clinic was due to run from 2 p.m. to 5 p.m. approximately. Therefore, the hospital authorities had deliberately arranged the session in such a way that some people would be waiting for three hours. The costs to Nicole were several, including the loss of time in which she could have been doing some of the many tasks that were pressing on her at home; the necessity to entertain her five-year-old daughter constantly for two hours to prevent her getting bored and restless; and the loss of face implied by the hospital authority's apparent attitude that it didn't matter if she was kept waiting for one, two or three hours.

Brandon, an electrician, was angry because he was asked to do too much at work. His boss asked in a very straightforward way, something like, 'Have you got time to fit in an extra call to a customer who needs their light switches sorting out?' and was quite prepared to take no for an answer; he could always ask another of the electricians. Nevertheless, Brandon was still angry because of the cost to him of the request. What was that cost? The way he saw it, he could choose one of two: either he suffered the cost of time, whereby he did an extra job that he couldn't really fit into his schedule; or he suffered the cost of guilt in turning down a straightforward request from his boss. Clearly Brandon needed to learn some deep assertiveness techniques, so that he could feel entitled to say 'no' without feeling guilty about it.

I have met a lot of people who get very angry and irritated when their partners contradict them in public. The cost here is usually loss of face – especially when the contradiction implies that the first speaker was telling a lie, even if only a harmless little lie to exaggerate and make more interesting an otherwise boring story. Errol, however, was driven wild by the very smallness of the contradiction. He gave me the example of an occasion when he and his wife were chatting with friends and he was recounting a story of something that had happened the previous Wednesday. As soon as he uttered the word 'Wednesday' his wife interrupted to say, 'No it wasn't, it was last Tuesday.' It is difficult to imagine that he could be made so angry by the cost of such an interruption: there is, after all, hardly any loss of face involved in mistaking a Tuesday for a Wednesday. Perhaps it was just a case of a simple irritant (having his flow of thought interrupted) – or possibly it was something different: a transgression.

Transgressions

A transgression involves the breaking of a rule. Possibly Errol held to the rule that husbands and wives don't contradict each other in public – not at all an unusual rule to have. Therefore, when that rule was broken, repeatedly, he got angry, increasingly.

Another very common rule that good friends and partners have is that confidences should not be broken. In other words, if your partner knows something about you purely by virtue of being your partner, then he or she should not go around telling other people about it. This might include intimate details about your health, your likes and dislikes, or simply something they know about your experiences or opinions which you would not share with anybody except your nearest and dearest. To break such confidences is almost universally viewed as a taboo, a major transgression – and one of the very quickest ways you can get on the wrong side of your partner.

Obviously, the example in Chapter 1 about the man who got angry with the youngster he caught trying to steal his car radio is also an example of a transgression. In that case the youngster was not just breaking a rule held by the man in question – he was breaking the law: a very formalised transgression.

These three categories are not mutually exclusive: there are many cases that cross the boundaries. For example, if your partner flirts with someone he or she finds attractive, that is normally viewed as a transgression; in other words, it is against the rules for many people. But it also involves a cost – loss of face, the impression that your partner is somehow dissatisfied with you and seeking consolation elsewhere. (Of course, this may not be true; but it is easily and often seen that way.)

Another cross-boundary example was the case of Lola's son, who accidentally dropped a mug on the floor and broke it. Perhaps it was, as his mother claimed, the cost of replacing the mug that made her angry; but, given that she could afford to do that without even noticing the price, that seems rather unlikely. A more probable explanation is that she was angry because he had transgressed an unspoken rule, namely that one takes a reasonable amount of care not to inconvenience others in the household. The 'sheer carelessness' was what made her angry.

Summary

- It is important to know the sorts of things which make you angry, because you will use this knowledge to benefit yourself later on.
- Typically, there are three categories of event that make people angry: irritants, costs and transgressions.
- There are plenty of irritants: people leaving doors open repeatedly, neighbours making a noise, even the way people eat or cough.
- Likewise, there are plenty of things that people do that have a cost for us: our children breaking things and the consequent financial cost; our partners contradicting us and costing us loss of face; having to do things unexpectedly, which costs us time.
- You, like everyone else, will have a set of rules that you expect other people to abide by. When someone breaks one of those rules, it is known as a transgression. When you spot a transgression, or think you have, the chances are you will be angry.
- Some things which make us angry straddle the boundaries between these categories. For example, a child breaking something may make us angry because of the cost involved in replacing it, but also because they have not, in our view, taken sufficient care.

4

Why am I not angry all the time?

It does seem that the world is absolutely crammed full with irritants, people doing things that have costs for us, and people breaking the rules we have made up for ourselves. So how come we are not in a permanent state of anger and rage?

Internal and external inhibitions

Remember Nicole, who took her youngster to the out-patient clinic at the hospital and was kept waiting for two hours? She described that event to me as one of the times she has been most angry in her life. There were various factors in the build-up. When she first got there, she saw the waiting room was very crowded, but thought perhaps there were quite a few doctors and nurses working, so that it would soon clear. Gradually she realised that, on the contrary, the queue was moving only very slowly; and when she got talking to some of the others there, she found that every one of them had a 2 p.m. appointment. That caused a major step change in her level of anger, from quite calm to 'pretty angry'. Not 'absolutely boiling', however: that came when, at around 3 p.m., the sole doctor and nurse who were in fact working at the clinic that day stopped to have their afternoon tea. And why shouldn't they? you ask; most of us perhaps take a short break in the afternoon, and they had been working hard. Why not, indeed; but it was the manner of their doing it that provoked Nicole. For they sat in the clinic room chatting to each other with the door wide open, so that all the patients could see them having their break – all the mothers (mostly) with their youngsters getting increasingly fretful while doctor and nurse only too visibly maintained their right to have a cup of tea. Not surprisingly, then, by the time Nicole took her little girl in to see the doctor she was purple with rage. So did she give the doctor a piece of her mind? No; she didn't say a word about it.

Now, this is amazing on the face of it, because if you talk to Nicole now, ten years after that event, she still begins seething at the recollection of it. She was *so angry*. And yet she simply didn't mention it when she got to see the doctor. Why could that be?

The short answer is: because of her *inhibitions*. It's not that Nicole is an 'inhibited' kind of person, just that there were inhibitions in action that held her back, some kind of self-control mechanism. We can probably guess the kind of thoughts that were going through her mind – things like: 'If I get on the wrong side of the doctor, will my youngster get the best treatment he is capable of providing?' Nicole, indeed, confirms that this is true, that is exactly the thought that was uppermost in her mind. But she also confesses to a secondary inhibition, namely: 'You just don't go around getting angry with doctors.' Rightly or wrongly, she held this as a rule for herself, a rule that held good even when she was so badly treated by a doctor.

That second inhibition ('you don't get angry with doctors') is termed an *internal* inhibition: in other words, it is an inhibition which exists entirely internally, in the mind. There is no external threat, like the police coming to arrest her, which would prevent her from being angry with the doctor, purely an internal rule she had for herself.

What about the first inhibition? The one which said maybe her child wouldn't get the very best treatment if she became angry with the doctor? Yes, that is an *external* inhibition, inasmuch as it was a fear of the consequences that stopped her venting her anger.

Let's look back now at the example in Chapter 1 where David came round the corner and saw a teenager smashing his car window and starting to take the stereo out. David caught the teenager, and, sitting astride him on the ground, described himself as being completely overwhelmed with anger against this boy who felt he could simply go and take things that didn't belong to him. So, now he had him on the ground, at his mercy, why didn't he throttle him or smash his head up and down against the pavement? Again, the answer is 'inhibitions': but were they internal or external? Was it the fear of being hauled off to court himself on a much more serious charge than theft, or was it some deeply ingrained rule that said you don't go smashing people's heads up and down on the pavement no matter what they've done?

Who knows? Probably a combination of the two. Either way, the episode certainly illustrates the power of such inhibitions because David clearly was, from his description, absolutely beside himself with rage.

Another example of the power of internal inhibitions – simple rules we make up for ourselves – came from a guy I was talking to recently who works in a bar. He described how one of his customers was arguing loudly with another and was going to hit him. The man who was about to be on the receiving end of the punch took a step back, raised his hands in a placatory gesture, and said, 'Hey, hey, hey . . . I'm over forty.' This remark, it seems, just put a pause in the proceedings while the would-be assailant checked his memory banks to see if there really was a rule against hitting people aged over forty. Interestingly, and no doubt much to the relief of the potential victim, by the time he had found that there wasn't really such a rule the moment had passed and he just stomped off.

Inhibitions as brakes on anger

Inhibitions, then, are in fact wonderful things – rather like the brakes on the car, they prevent us from going too far too fast. Later on in this book we are going to see how you can use inhibitions to your own benefit, so it is a good idea right now to get used to the idea that inhibitions are necessary and helpful mechanisms built right into the structure of our brains. It is also worth emphasising that referring to 'inhibitions' in this sense is different from referring to somebody as 'inhibited', as a term of criticism. What we often mean in that context is that the person is constrained from displaying any emotion, not just anger, so that they may appear cold, detached, self-absorbed and unable to 'let themselves go'. But in the context of keeping our angry reactions in check, inhibitions – both internal and external – are just what we want.

Let's take one example of somebody who had not developed his inhibitions strongly enough – someone to whom, as a result, I was talking inside a prison. Terry recounted how one night he was standing at a bar, having a drink with a friend. He thinks he had probably had four or five pints of beer by the time the following incident took place. He says he was just lifting his pint mug to his mouth when somebody nearby jogged his elbow, with the result that a good amount of beer went not into his mouth but all over his face and chest. The next thing he knew, Terry had smashed his beer mug against the bar and pushed it into the man's face – thereby, of course, inflicting very severe injury indeed. The net result of those few seconds for Terry was a five-year prison sentence. It was a great pity for both men that the assailant had not worked on developing his inhibitions. Again, those inhibitions could have been external (I'll end up in prison, I'll be thrown out of the bar, the police will be called) or internal (it's not right to go around attacking people).

For most people, of course, the consequences of having undeveloped inhibitions are less dramatic than this: just living a life which is impaired year after year by upsetting other people! So, there are immense benefits to be gained from learning about inhibitions and all the other techniques that we will cover later. For now it is sufficient to know about them and to know how important they are.

What holds us back?

Now we have seen how inhibitions operate, perhaps we can work out what holds people back in each of the situations we have looked at.

- Why doesn't the person who hears loud music from next door immediately go round and complain angrily? *Answer:* internal inhibition: 'It's right to be tolerant towards your neighbours'; external inhibition: 'If I do that he will probably come round here complaining as soon as I make a noise, and he will probably go around badmouthing me to all our other neighbours.'
- Why didn't Aisha get angrier with her noisy-eating husband? *Answer:* internal inhibition: 'I must try and limit the amount of complaining I do, this is only a small thing'; external inhibition: 'I have probably got some bad habits too,

so if I complain about his eating, he will probably start complaining about all the things I do
that annoy him.'

- When people coughing during my talks used to
annoy me, why did I not get angry with them
and tell them to shut up or clear off? *Answer:*
internal inhibition 'I shouldn't speak rudely to
people who have come to hear me talk'; external inhibition: 'If I do that then there will be
an icy-cold atmosphere for the remainder of the
three days while everybody else is frightened to
death of accidentally coughing.'

- Why did Errol not snap back angrily when
his wife contradicted him in public? *Answer:*
internal inhibition: 'You don't wash your dirty
linen in public'; external inhibition: 'People will
think worse of me if I do that.'

- Why did Brandon, the electrician who was
asked to do too many jobs, not say 'no' to his
boss straight away? *Answer:* external inhibition:
his boss might think worse of him and, come
the time for redundancies . . .

Summary

- The ability to inhibit or control our anger is a very important ability to have. It is by no means a good idea to be 'uninhibited' where expressing our anger is concerned.
- This is not to say that you should never express your anger; rather, that you will be able to control your anger. As we saw in Chapter 1, irritable and over-angry people are those whose reaction is out of proportion to the situation that provokes the reaction.
- Inhibitions are like the brakes of a car: sometimes they stop the car moving, but often they simply ensure the car moves at an appropriate pace.
- Inhibitions are of two main types: internal and external.
- Internal inhibitions are the thoughts and moral guidelines we have for ourselves.
- External inhibitions are based on the awareness of the consequences that would take place if your response is judged to be out of proportion to the provocation.

Optional exercises

Think of a time you recently managed to control your temper. What helped you do that? Was it internal inhibitions (rules you have for yourself), external inhibitions (fear of the consequences) or something else entirely?

What was special about that time that made you able to control your temper on that occasion when you have trouble doing so on other occasions (assuming you do, given you're reading this book)?

5

Constructing a system to explain irritability and anger

The 'leaky bucket'

If we can put all that we have worked out so far into a diagram, it will help us predict when we are going to be irritable or angry and, more to the point, prevent it happening. So let's have a look at Figure 5.1, overleaf, which summarises what we have said so far about Nicole's case.

This is actually a particularly interesting example, because many people ask: 'What happens to the anger?' In other words, a lot of people assume that unless you 'let it out' then your anger just builds up inside you and ends up harming you in some unspecified way. So they let it out. The trouble is that 'let it out' is a euphemism; what it often means is getting angry with people, maybe shouting and swearing at them, maybe saying things that hurt the other person, and – what do you think – if we do this it usually doesn't improve

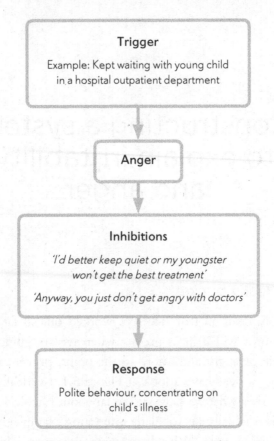

Figure 5.1 Kept waiting in hospital

things for us. The good news is that we don't have to do it; nothing bad happens if we refrain from shouting, swearing etc. What happens is that the anger inside us just gradually dissipates – it leaks away. The best analogy is a leaky bucket full of water. The bucket was full to overflowing in Nicole's case, she was very angry indeed. Nevertheless, over time, all that anger just gradually seeped away, just as water seeps out of a leaky bucket, and now in the ordinary course of things she doesn't give it a thought.

(It is worth noting that there are some emotions where it is good to be open and honest about them – to 'let them out' – because it leads to a better understanding between people, and if you are depressed or anxious for, example, it may lead to you obtaining support. Anger is different: letting it out usually means what we just described – shouting and saying bad things, and it rarely works well for us or anybody else.)

The key concept is *doing what you think is appropriate in the situation.* In this case the mother judged that her behaviour was indeed appropriate as her child might well have not received the best treatment if she had made a fuss. So, even in retrospect, she still judges that she did right. By the same token, we get angry with ourselves when, in retrospect, we think we did not behave correctly. Again, the important concept is behaving in proportion to the situation, doing what you think is right in the particular situation. (Later on, we will look at why our judgement sometimes goes haywire so that on occasion we let ourselves down very badly.)

Figure 5.2 shows the same model applied to a different situation. The key difference is that here the inhibitions weren't strong enough to control the level of anger experienced by Lola. The anger therefore simply overcame her inhibitions and produced a response of 'ranting and raving'.

Actually, this does Lola a slight disservice. Certainly this is the way she described the incident – that she simply 'lost

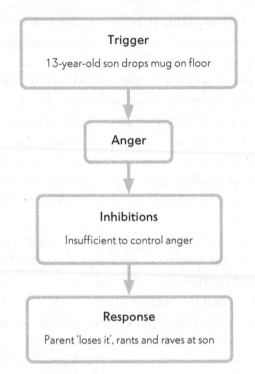

Figure 5.2 Mug breaks on floor

it', in other words, simply lost all control. But if that were really true, why did she not pick up the carving knife (they were in the kitchen, after all) and stab her son fifty times?

Ponder point

Try to answer this question: Lola says that she 'lost it' in that she was completely unable to control her temper and 'ranted and raved' at her son, which she very much regrets

54

but was totally unable to help herself. That can't be true can it? *If she was totally unable to help herself why didn't she do something more drastic like stab her son to death?* (For a suggested answer, see the end of this chapter.)

When the bucket overflows

Let's pursue this line of thought a little further by considering the case of Omar and a door left open in a bar. Omar was sitting near the door with his two friends, and it was a cold winter evening outside. What happened is described in Figure 5.3.

On the face of it, Figure 5.3 gives us an accurate representation of what happened. However, the exact situation is that this was the fifth time the door had been left slightly ajar. On each of the previous four occasions, some extra anger had been tipped into the bucket. So, by the time person number five comes along and adds his ladleful to the bucket, the whole thing is brim-full and ready to overflow – and Omar gives 'person number five' the whole bucket full of anger. Omar said when he was telling me the story that the 'victim' was quite a small man. What if he had been six feet three, built to match, and a 6th dan judo black belt? Do you think that would have strengthened Omar's inhibitions? Most people feel inhibited about picking a fight with someone twice their size.

This concept of anger building up to the point where it overflows is an important one. Adam, a senior salesman, told me the how he was repeatedly away from home on

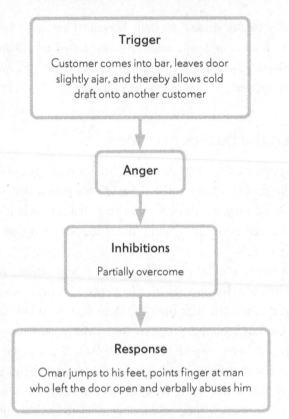

Trigger

Customer comes into bar, leaves door
slightly ajar, and thereby allows cold
draft onto another customer

Anger

Inhibitions

Partially overcome

Response

Omar jumps to his feet, points finger at man
who left the door open and verbally abuses him

Figure 5.3 Door left open in bar

business, jetting around the world to various exotic destinations for weeks on end. While he was away his attractive young wife Lisa took to having one affair after another. Gradually Adam became suspicious and, after he had confronted her several times, Lisa admitted what had been going on. Though obviously hurt, Adam thought he could cope and put it to his wife that so long as she told him everything he would be prepared to make a fresh start if she would too. So, through the course of the evening, Lisa confessed to the four affairs she had had. She went slowly and tactfully, and Adam was able gradually to come to terms with what had happened. They went to bed, resolved that they could put it all behind them and make a fresh start.

But Lisa had remembered a fifth affair, and when they woke up the following morning, in the spirit of making a clean breast of it, she confessed it. For Adam, this was enough to make the bucket overflow, and they divorced.

What makes you angry?

By now you should be able to start making a tentative analysis of what makes *you* irritable and angry.

- You may well be able to identify several triggers; for most people there is more than one thing that makes them angry.
- You may even be able to quantify the amount of anger that each trigger typically produces, perhaps using a 10-point scale where 10 out of 10 is the angriest you could ever be!
- Maybe you can identify what inhibitions come into play: both your internal inhibitions (the personal morality and rules you have for your own behaviour) and the external inhibitions (consequences that may befall you if you overreact).

- You may also be able to reflect upon the various responses you have made in the past when these triggers have set off your anger.

There is no need to do all that at this stage unless you want to; later on we will look at how to analyse these elements carefully, and what to do once you've analysed them. It can be interesting and rewarding to do so. But for now it may be useful to consider the kinds of questions we will be asking.

Summary

- We can construct a realistic model which explains how anger and our subsequent reactions to it come about.
- It is well worth doing this because we can then analyse our own actions, and those of others. Armed with this awareness, we can then intervene to lessen the anger we experience – and, moreover, to alter the responses we produce. It is those responses that people normally refer to as our 'irritability' or 'anger'.
- We will be developing this model as we go through the book. The key headings so far are: the trigger (what triggers our anger); the

anger itself (which can gradually build up, like increasing amounts of water being poured into a bucket); inhibitions (which stop us constantly giving vent to our anger); and the response (which can range from nothing at all, when we completely control our anger, through to catastrophic responses when we totally fail to control it.)

- Importantly, there is no need to 'let our anger out'. Very often, 'letting our anger out' simply makes it worse. Better to let it slowly seep away, like water running out from a leaky bucket.

Suggested answer to the Ponder point

If Lola was totally unable to help herself why didn't she do something more drastic like stab her son to death?

Maybe Lola doesn't see 'ranting and raving' at her son as being nearly as bad as stabbing him to death. Now you and I might say, 'Well of course she doesn't, it isn't nearly as bad'. And yet, when you talk to Lola she is adamant that she no more wants to 'lose it' with her son than she wants to stab him. And yet this can't be true can it, because she does the former but not the latter.

I think the two actions are coded in Lola's brain as quite different. Stabbing is coded as something that 'Of course I wouldn't do that, I would never do that, no mother would ever do that', whereas losing it is coded as 'This is something I really don't want to do, I hate myself for doing it'.

What do you think would happen if Lola managed to recode ranting and raving at her son as 'Of course I wouldn't do that, I would never do that, no mother would ever do that'?

6

Why don't other people feel angry at the things that bug me? Appraisals and judgements

If we can really plot things out just as neatly and tidily as described in the previous chapter, then you would think that what triggers one person's anger would trigger the same response in another person. And, to a large extent, this is true. Most people, for example, don't like other people shouting and swearing at them. It makes them angry; it is a trigger for their anger. Most people don't like other folk stealing from them; that too is a trigger for their anger. Most people don't like sitting in interminable traffic jams. That too makes most people angry, to a greater or lesser degree. But it is also true that people respond quite differently to some triggers. For instance, one person may get angry at the sight of teenagers playing football outside his house, whereas another may view it as part of community life.

Seeing things differently

And that is the point. It is all to do with *how we view* the event in question. If we take a hostile view of it, then it will indeed become a trigger for our anger. If we view it tolerantly and benignly, it won't.

This is not to say that we should view everything in a tolerant and benign way. As we shall see later, anger can be very useful and productive. Nevertheless, for the time being, let us just look at how things normally work.

- How come one person kept waiting in a hospital outpatient clinic became really angry whereas another person didn't? Answer: because the first person viewed it as inconsiderate and arrogant to schedule everybody in for a 2 p.m. appointment in a clinic which lasts three hours, and believes that people should show proper consideration for each other. The second person says, 'It's just one of those things', and expects no better from people.

- Why does one man get intensely irritated by teenagers playing soccer outside his house, while his next-door neighbour doesn't? Answer: because the first person sees it not only as lacking in consideration because of the amount of noise it creates, but also as a symbol of living in a more downmarket area than he would wish to.

The second person sees it as part and parcel of living in a friendly, lively community.

- Why does one man sitting by a bar door get up and confront the person who left it ajar, whereas the others aren't bothered? Answer: because that man believed that each person who left the door open was doing it as a deliberate provocation and felt that he was losing face in front of the other drinkers. The other two felt there was no offence meant – just that people coming into a bar are normally more concerned about getting a drink than closing the door.

- Why does one woman get angry about her husband eating in a very noisy way, while the same thing doesn't bother thousands of others at all? Answer: because she sees it as a symbol of the difference between their backgrounds, a constant suggestion that they really should not be married at all; for her, it epitomises the difference between them. For others, how much noise a person makes when they eat has no significance.

- Why did I at one stage get particularly uptight about people coughing during my talks, whereas later on it didn't bother me? Answer: because initially I thought that they might not be paying me enough attention, or even be deliberately provoking me, whereas later I felt they were doing well to come to the course when they could be off sick.

- Why does one parent get angry when their son drops a mug on the floor and it breaks, whereas another simply says, 'Never mind', and gets him to sweep it up? Answer: because the first person sees it as wilful carelessness and a disregard of how much it costs to replace things, whereas the second realises that they can easily afford to buy another mug without noticing it.

- Why does one man get angry when his partner contradicts him in public whereas another one doesn't? Because the first man views the contradiction as saying to everybody present that his wife doesn't respect him, whereas the second man views it as 'just the way she is'.

- Why does one mother get angry when she finds her daughter taking a leisurely bath whereas another doesn't? Answer: because the first mother said to herself that her daughter was only having a bath to avoid tidying her room, whereas the second mother was pleased to see her daughter taking good care of herself.

- Why does one father get angry enough with his son to hit him when he sees he has not completed his homework, whereas another father doesn't? Answer: Because the first father says that his son is a lazy good-for-nothing so-and-so who is trying to pull the wool over his eyes, whereas the second father says that any normal twelve-year-old is bound to be more interested in watching television than doing his homework.

. . . and so on. In other words, it is not so much the trigger *in itself* that produces the anger; it is what goes through the person's mind when prompted by the trigger.

Appraisals and Judgements

Returning to our model as set out in Chapter 4, we can now extend it to apply to three of the cases we have looked at, as shown in Figures 6.1–6.3.

This one extra box we have put into our model, headed 'Appraisal/Judgement', is a very important one. It means that no longer are we at the mercy of events, or 'triggers'. Now we can see that it is we ourselves who can decide what to make of these events, how to appraise or judge them. It is our appraisal or judgement which will determine whether we will get angry and to what degree. What is more, we can actually *check out our appraisal* with that of others. For example, the man in the bar could have said to his two friends: 'Do you think these people are deliberately leaving the door open to annoy us . . . do you think everyone is laughing at us behind our backs?' Whereupon, in all probability, he would have been reassured that this was

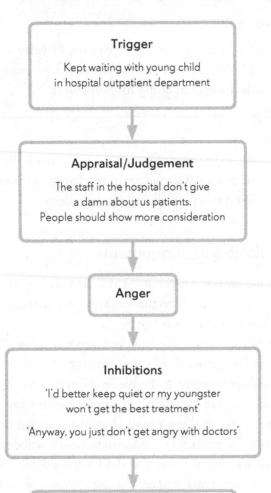

Figure 6.1 Kept waiting in hospital

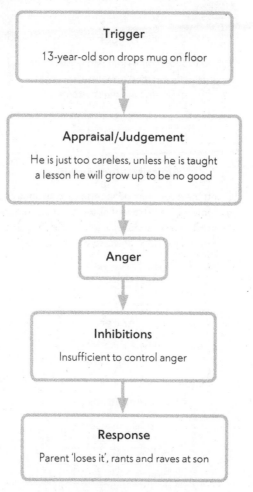

Figure 6.2 Mug breaks on floor

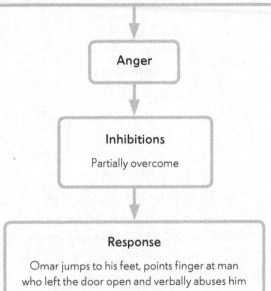

Trigger

Customer comes into bar, leaves door slightly ajar, and thereby allows cold draft onto another customer

Appraisal/Judgement

He's left the door open deliberately just to annoy me and show me up in front of all the other customers. If I don't react everybody's going to be laughing behind my back, or worse still, to my face

Anger

Inhibitions

Partially overcome

Response

Omar jumps to his feet, points finger at man who left the door open and verbally abuses him

Figure 6.3 Door left open in bar

not so, that the door was just not working properly, and this might have prevented him from getting angry.

There is an important point here. Many people think that because they believe something is true, it necessarily *is* true: for instance, in this case, 'Because I believe he left the door open to annoy me, it is true that he did indeed leave the door open to annoy me.' This is very far from being the case; but it is an easy trap to fall into until we get used to questioning our judgements and checking them out with other people.

Summary

- This chapter has added just one more box to our model, but it is an important box.
- That important box, 'Appraisal/Judgement', goes between 'Trigger' and 'Anger', and may totally prevent the trigger producing anger.
- Later, we will look at ways of examining and altering our appraisals/judgements. For the time being, it is enough to know that simply because we think something is true, that does not actually make it true.
- We are now working towards a comprehensive model with which to examine events that make us angry out of proportion to what one would reasonably expect.

Suggested project

There is a key observation in this chapter, namely 'Just because we think something is true, doesn't make it true.' So just because we're convinced that someone did something deliberately to annoy us it doesn't mean that they did! So the project I suggest is:

1. Try to notice a time where you are making an assumption about a situation
2. Check out your assumption with someone else.

Curiously, I can give you an example. I was having lunch with two friends in a very nice London restaurant – the kind of restaurant you only go to occasionally. Just behind us was a serving station with an attentive high-level waiter standing there. So far so good except that it was close to us and he was drumming his fingers on the wood of the table. Just as in the chapter examples, I was getting irritated by it. In fact, more than that, I thought it was definitely irritating – it wasn't just me, it would be irritating to anyone. So, I checked it out with the other two and they said, 'What drumming . . . Oh *that* drumming . . . No I hadn't noticed.' It was as well that I did because their saying that changed my appraisal: if they weren't bothered why should I be?

So the suggested project is to see if you can spot any situation similar to that happening to you – a situation where you are making an assumption you are so convinced about that you think it is a fact rather than an assumption. Then to check out the way you're seeing it with someone else who is present. It can be very interesting.

7

Why isn't everybody irritated by the same things? Beliefs

This sounds like pretty much the same question we asked in Chapter 6, and in a sense it is. But bear with me, because there is a significant difference. You will remember that, in Chapter 6, we asked the question: 'Why do some triggers make me angry but not other people, and vice versa?' and the answer was: Because you might appraise and judge the situation one way, and other people might appraise and judge it another way. The question we are really addressing in this chapter, to put it in its fullest form, is: 'Why do I appraise and judge a situation in one way, whereas somebody else might appraise and judge it in quite a different way?'

Beliefs

So, how come you appraise and judge a situation one way while some other people appraise and judge it in another way? The answer is: 'Because of the basic beliefs we have all developed over the years.' These beliefs can be of several different kinds, for example:

- Beliefs about how other people are, what the world is like, even about how we compare with other people.
- Beliefs about how people are meant to behave, how people 'learn lessons', what's important in life, and so on.
- Beliefs about how other people would see a particular situation, including possibly how a jury in a court of law would see it.

How do these beliefs fit in with the model we developed in the previous chapter? Clearly, our beliefs are going to influence:

- Our judgement and appraisal of the trigger.
- Our anger.
- Our inhibitions.
- Our feelings of anger.
- Our response.

So now our model has another element in it, as shown in Figure 7.1.

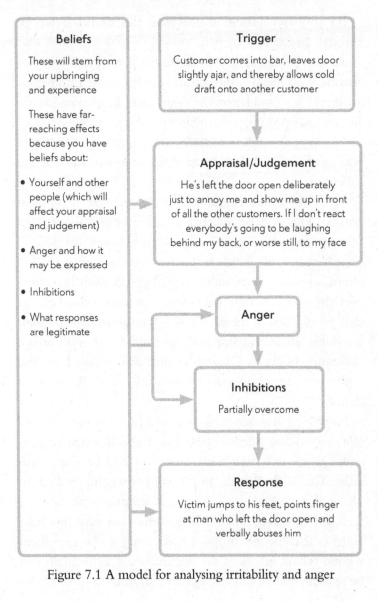

Figure 7.1 A model for analysing irritability and anger

It's probably easiest to see how this works if we go through an example or two.

As above, regarding the man in the bar, sitting with two friends, who finally jumps up and confronts the fifth person who comes in and leaves the door open: How come it was he who jumped up, rather than one of his two friends?

Working through our model, we can see that the trigger was just the same for all three of them: so that can't be the difference.

What about the appraisal or judgement each of them makes? This will be affected by their beliefs about what other people are like. If one of them believes that people, generally, are 'all selfish bastards who don't give a damn about anyone except themselves' he will probably inter- pret the situation differently from someone who believes that people 'are all basically good, though sometimes their goodness needs bringing out'. So maybe that was the key difference between Omar (the one who jumped up and confronted the newcomer) and Carlos and Ryan (who didn't).

Now we can move on to our next box, marked 'Anger'. We can see that, primed by his beliefs about people in gen- eral, Omar's brain is already more likely to be angry than either Carlos' or Ryan's; and it will be 'recommending' to Omar that he makes a response in keeping with how he feels. At this stage, too, beliefs come into play. If Omar believes that 'people only learn anything if you give them a good telling off' then the chances are that his brain will be recommending something different from those of Carlos and Ryan, who believe for the most part that 'the only way people learn anything is when they are allowed to sit down and think things through'.

From here we move on to 'Inhibitions'. By now we can see that Omar, who thinks that people are 'all selfish bastards who don't give a damn about anyone except themselves' and that 'people only learn anything if you give them a good telling off', is already thinking in terms of a pretty hostile response. But possibly his inhibitions will tone it down. If he believes that 'you don't show your anger in public', that might keep him under control. Equally, if he believes that 'if you confront somebody they are liable to attack you,' then that too will restrain him, so long as the person leaving the door open looks like he can handle himself. On the other hand, if he believes that 'if somebody deliberately provokes you then you've got to show them who's boss', this is unlikely to do much to keep his anger in check.

Finally, then, we come to his response. We can see that beliefs are going to play a part here. If he believes that 'It's all right thumping somebody but you don't ever use a weapon', his response is clearly going to be of a different order than if he believes that 'If you're going to pick a fight with somebody you have to be tooled up.'

So we can see in this example that the beliefs Omar holds are going to affect him at every stage. And these beliefs are *nothing to do with the situation in question*; they are beliefs he holds day in, day out. So if Omar wanted to radically alter the way he is, the way he feels and the way he reacts, he could work on his beliefs, perhaps bring them a bit closer to those of Carlos and Ryan. We'll see how later on.

What about the two mothers and their daughters in the bath? One mother, Amy, got really angry with her daughter because she wasn't tidying her room. Amy's next-door neighbour, Lin, also has fairly young children and she has always reacted differently to them in the face of stress. So let's have a look at how our model would compare Amy and Lin. Again, the trigger or situation would have to be just the same: how would Lin react if her twelve-year-old had been resolutely not tidying her room, and how would this compare with Amy's reaction?

Let's have a look at the judgement or appraisal that each would make in the face of this event. Amy's judgement is influenced by the fact that she believes her daughter 'deliberately does everything she can to annoy me'. Lin, on the other hand, believes that 'Children don't annoy you deliberately, but they are naturally selfish and only lose that as they get older'. Amy, therefore, is inclined to see her twelve-year-old's behaviour as deliberate defiance, designed to provoke her; Lin, on the other hand, views her daughter's similar behaviour as a piece of thoughtlessness typical of a child of that age. As a result, Amy is inclined to be angry, Lin much less so.

As a result of this belief, Amy's angry brain is already recommending some kind of angry response. Unfortunately, Amy also believes that 'You get nowhere by spoiling kids', with the corresponding implication that 'a firm hand', either metaphorically or literally, is what is required. Lin thinks differently. Even when she does get angry (which, you will be pleased to hear, she does sometimes) her basic belief is that 'Children need a good example set for them'. So, while she doesn't mind confronting issues with her children, and them knowing that she is angry and hearing it in her voice, she does try hard not to 'shout and scream at them', and certainly doesn't believe in smacking them.

What about inhibitions? Amy believes that if her neighbours hear her 'going over the top' in terms of shouting or smacking her youngster they will report her to social services. She says this is one of the main things that makes her able sometimes to control her temper. Lin believes that it is simply not right to shout and scream at young children, and certainly not to hit them.

In terms of response, Amy thinks that 'A good smack never did anyone any harm', while Lin believes that 'Adults hitting children is simply bullying'.

Beliefs and behaviour

One of the interesting points raised by the example of Amy and Lin is that it doesn't matter whether beliefs are right or not; they still influence the behaviour of the person who holds them. For instance, Amy may be correct in believing that 'Kids do all they can to deliberately annoy you' and Lin may be wrong in believing that 'Children are just selfish by nature and grow out of it eventually'. It really doesn't matter who is right and who is wrong: both are heavily influenced by their own beliefs. You sometimes even see the paradoxical situation where Lin's child may be annoying her quite deliberately but, because Lin believes what she does, she not only leads a calmer life but also sets a better example for her child.

Let's look at another example, this time involving flirting. Ella and Lemy live on a new housing development, and Lemy has quite serious problems with jealousy. Michelle and Jamie are another young couple who live nearby. Ella and Michelle are good friends and are very similar in many respects. Unlike Lemy, however, Jamie has no problems with jealousy.

On several occasions Lemy and Jamie have faced more or less the same 'trigger'. From time to time both couples find themselves at the same party – in fact, very often they will actually all go to the party together. Both Ella and Michelle are warm, friendly and extrovert young women who like to have an uninhibited time simply in terms of dancing, drinking and feeling the pleasure of having friends around them. Lemy and Jamie appraise these 'triggers' in quite different ways. Lemy believes that if a woman is married then she shouldn't be showing any interest in any other man, and this is what he perceives Ella as doing. Jamie, on the other hand, believes that it is only natural for women to show an interest in men and vice versa. He simply believes that if you are married then 'You shouldn't take it any further than the interest stage'. So, as a result of the same events, Lemy becomes angry whereas Jamie doesn't. Lemy's angry brain is recommending to him an angry response, whereas Jamie's is not.

In terms of inhibitions, Lemy believes that it is wrong to hit anybody, and certainly somebody you love, so even though angry he will not respond that way. (Interestingly, Jamie is not totally averse to getting into fights; he does not believe that is totally wrong. Fortunately, however, he rarely becomes angry.) Lemy also believes that if he 'addresses the issue head on' then (a) Ella will think he is a 'wimp' for being jealous, and (b) this will put a dampener on the fun they might have at any future party.

In terms of responses, Lemy believes it is wrong to hit people, so that is ruled out. He also believes it is undesirable to shout or to address the issue head on, so he tends not to do this. His beliefs about sulking, however, are not quite so negative, so that is what he tends to end up doing. Jamie, on the other hand, believes that 'Sulking is something women do', so even when angry doesn't tend to respond like that. It is clear from these examples that our beliefs can have an all-pervasive effect on us – not just on irritability and anger but on every aspect of our feelings and emotions: jealousy, anxiety, depression, anything you care to mention.

Beliefs and other people

Once a year my mother and I go off on two or three days' holiday, just the two of us (my family stays behind and has a bit of respite). A couple of years ago we found ourselves in Paris, in an extremely nice hotel which we could never have afforded had it not been for a special offer at the travel agent. Anyway, once there, we look around for what to do.

Tickets available from the hotel include an evening at the Moulin Rouge which is, as you know, a kind of review bar for tourists. It looks good, and of all the attractions on offer it is the only one we have heard of. The only snag is that it is expensive: I think it was about 120 euros per person for the evening – that's about £100 or $150. However, this (it seems) includes everything: dinner, drinks, review, the lot. So we sign up, and the next evening off we go. The Moulin Rouge consists of a big stage on which a lot of girls strut their stuff – and an even bigger area where about five million tourists eat their dinners at tables crammed more closely together than you have ever seen before. We are given a terrific table, right next to the stage, are given complimentary drinks shortly followed by the first course of our dinner, and sit back for a good evening. As the show starts, I notice a very small card sitting on the table, pick it up and just manage to read what it says in the gloom. My hazy brain does a slow translation: 'minimum drinks order 200 euros per person'. I am stunned. Not only having paid handsomely for our two tickets, we are now faced with having to pay another substantial sum for drinks. I am not even sure I have got that much money on me. Everywhere I look I see twenty-stone bouncers, and begin to realise the true meaning of the phrase 'tourist trap'.

My mother is pretty engrossed in the show. I am feeling sort of nauseous, and, even from the inside, can tell I must look glazed. The third act finishes and there is a gap before the band starts up to herald the fourth act. At this point I mention, calmly of course, that there is a card on the table that says there is a minimum drinks order which will bankrupt us.

And this is where beliefs come in. Me, I believe that all big cities are the same and that if you go to a tourist trap then you expect to get trapped. My mother, she has had good holidays in France so, quick as a flash, she says: 'No, it's all right, French people are nice' – without taking her eyes off the stage. It is a simple belief, deeply embedded, and has ramifications for a thousand and one situations that might arise in France. (And, thank goodness, she was right: the card's strictures didn't apply to us.)

Not long after the Moulin Rouge experience, I came across another example of an extended version of 'French people are nice'. I was walking along a promenade in a quiet coastal resort, and coming towards me was a man of about twenty-five who clearly had significant learning difficulties. He had a rucksack which was causing him some trouble: he had managed to get it properly hooked over one shoulder, but the other side was sort of pinning his arm halfway behind him. This posture will be familiar to anyone who has ever tried to put a rucksack on; and it's much more easily sorted out by someone else than by the wearer. So this man simply walked up and stood in front of me without saying a word; and I sorted out his rucksack.

What does that say about this man's beliefs about other people? *'Other people are nice.'* So nice, in fact, that if you are having trouble with your rucksack, all you have to do is go and stand in front of a random person and he or she will sort you out. You don't even have to say anything!

So, not only do underlying beliefs influence just about every moment of your life, but doing a bit of work on your beliefs can pay off handsomely. We'll look at how to do this later on in the book.

Where do beliefs come from?

You might be wondering where our beliefs come from. Well, clearly they come from our experiences. Many of them come from early experience (our childhood, school and upbringing) and are never revised. Sometimes, for example, people are taught as children that everybody in the world is out for what they can get, so you have to watch your back. Others, although they are not explicitly taught such lessons, pick them up for themselves through observing others. Equally, many people are taught as children that 'people are basically good', or have had the sort of upbringing which has led them to believe that this is the case, whether or not it was spelt out for them.

On the basis of these 'mega-beliefs' we make rules for ourselves. For instance, if I believe that everyone is out for what they can get, I will have a series of sub-beliefs along the lines of 'I must keep my wits about me', 'You have to watch everybody like a hawk or they'll take advantage of you', and 'If you give someone an inch they'll take a mile'. Equally, if I believe that people are basically good I will have a series of sub-beliefs along the lines of 'We must trust each other in order to flourish', 'The best place to relax is in the company of others', and so on.

Summary

- We set out in this chapter to answer the question of why a particular situation would irritate one person and not another.

- We came to the conclusion that it is to do with our beliefs about ourselves, other people, the nature of the world, how people are meant to behave and how we are meant to behave.

- These beliefs are developed over the years through our experiences and observations, often based on the things we are told when we are young.

- We found that our beliefs also underlie our inhibitions. Some people believe that you shouldn't ever hit anybody, even if it's called 'smacking'. Other people believe you mustn't hit anybody unless it's someone much smaller than yourself, like your child. Other people believe that it's wrong to shout. Other people believe that it's right to talk things through with people even if they are very young. Other people believe that to set a good example is very important. All these beliefs will form part of our internal inhibitions. Others are much more constrained by the likely results of their actions, so believe that it is ill-advised to pick a fight with somebody bigger and fitter than you, as you're likely to get hurt; these beliefs form part of their external inhibitions.

- People even have beliefs about the kind of responses it's okay to make. Some people believe that an obviously aggressive response is inappropriate, but sulking would be okay; and so on.

- All this knowledge about beliefs and their influence forms another important area that we will be able to use to our benefit when we come to Part Two of this book.

Exercise

As you've been reading this chapter you maybe identified with one or other of the many beliefs expressed by the various characters who featured. The exercise I suggest is that you write down (or, at least, bring very clearly to mind) the belief you most identified with. Then I suggest you spend a couple of minutes pondering how that belief has affected the way you feel or act, and also wondering how things might be different if you believed something quite different.

8

Why am I sometimes more irritable than at other times? Moods

Up to now we've concentrated largely on the question 'Why do some people get angry more easily than other people?' And we've come up with lots of answers – or at least, we could work out lots of answers for lots of different situations if we wanted to by going through our model. Some of the answers might be as follows:

- Charlie gets more angry than Ben because Charlie finds himself in more anger-making situations than Ben does.
- Laura gets more angry than Magda because Laura tends to judge and appraise situations differently from the way Magda does.
- Kelly gets more angry than Erin because her inhibitions aren't so well developed.

- Barry seems to get more angry than Kyle because Barry will countenance more hostile responses than Kyle does. For example, Barry will shout and threaten while Kyle tends to sulk.
- Rachel gets more angry than Sara because Rachel believes that other people are basically a self-centred lot who can't be trusted, so she tends to misinterpret some situations.

. . . and so on.

So, we can now make some more informed and reliable judgements about why some people get more angry than others, or seem to be more angry than others (because of the way they respond when they are angry). And this is good, because if we want to be one of those people who is angry less often we can already see that there are going to be some very powerful things we can achieve. We have a nice model which we can apply systematically in your own particular case.

Moods

But for many people it is the *variation* in their irritability that really concerns them: in other words, some days they feel really irritable, other days they don't. If you are one of these people then you will know that this variation causes major problems for people around you, because they never know 'what mood you're going to be in'. So they can never relax properly with you, and that in turn means that the feelings of intimacy and closeness that would otherwise develop between you and them simply don't have a chance to take root.

Moreover, you will also know that this causes major problems for yourself – not just in how it impairs the intimacy of relationships, but also because you continually feel as though you have 'let yourself down'. If you have these big variations in irritability you will sometimes look back on things you did yesterday, or even earlier on today, and feel embarrassed or ashamed by them. For, although they seemed perfectly sensible and justifiable at the time, now you can see that you were being excessively irritable – you were in 'a bad mood'. (Actually, they don't always seem that sensible at the time; maybe you know when you're feeling irritable, and that's a very bad feeling. The trouble is that it seems very difficult to 'snap out of it' at the time, and indeed it is.)

The good news is that there are all sorts of things that we can do to keep ourselves in a 'stable mood'. But first we need to focus on the key concept of 'mood'.

In terms of our model, like 'Beliefs', mood influences all four of the major boxes from 'Appraisal/Judgement' downwards, so that the model now looks like Figure 8.1.

Lots of people have trouble with their moods, as illustrated by the following table (Table 8.1).

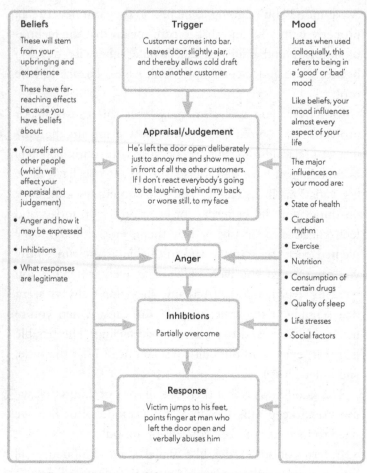

Beliefs

These will stem from your upbringing and experience

These have far-reaching effects because you have beliefs about:

- Yourself and other people (which will affect your appraisal and judgement)

- Anger and how it may be expressed

- Inhibitions

- What responses are legitimate

Trigger

Customer comes into bar, leaves door slightly ajar, and thereby allows cold draft onto another customer

Mood

Just as when used colloquially, this refers to being in a 'good' or 'bad' mood

Like beliefs, your mood influences almost every aspect of your life

The major influences on your mood are:

- State of health
- Circadian rhythm
- Exercise
- Nutrition
- Consumption of certain drugs
- Quality of sleep
- Life stresses
- Social factors

Appraisal/Judgement

He's left the door open deliberately just to annoy me and show me up in front of all the other customers. If I don't react everybody's going to be laughing behind my back, or worse still, to my face

Anger

Inhibitions

Partially overcome

Response

Victim jumps to his feet, points finger at man who left the door open and verbally abuses him

Figure 8.1 A model for analysing irritability and anger

Table 8.1 Good Moods and Bad Moods

Good Moods and Bad Moods		
Situation	How Tim sees things when he's in a good mood	How Tim sees things when he's in a bad mood
Husband eating noisily	Doesn't notice	'Totally unbearable'
Children dropping and breaking things	'Accidents will happen – I've broken enough things myself in my time'	'Drives me completely mad – it's just pure carelessness'
Waiting for two hours in an outpatient clinic with child	Likely to see it as a chance to get to know the other mums	Storms straight into the clinic room and has it out with the doctor there and then
Husband 'telling all and sundry what they've been talking about'	Never takes a positive view of her husband talking about things she regards as 'between them'; however, 'best just to leave it'	'The last straw – I just feel like walking out on him at that very moment'
Children are disobedient	It's no use getting het up about what your kids do, there's no changing them'	'I wonder why I ever had them'

It's clear from these few examples that anybody who is in a remotely similar situation to the above good/bad moods will be having a great deal of trouble making sense of their life. One day they're up, the next day they're down. One day they're laughing and joking with people; another day they're snapping their heads off. Worse than that, it can vary from one half-hour to another. So what kind of things do we have to watch out for to keep our mood steady? Some of the main factors are:

- Illness: mental illnesses (such as depression) or physical illnesses (such as viral infections) can both disrupt your mood.
- Routine: it is very important to maintain a fairly consistent routine in terms of times of eating and sleeping, to maintain a steady 'circadian rhythm'. Otherwise you find yourself in a permanent state of 'jetlag', which is very disruptive.
- Exercise: humans are built for activity, and during phases when we don't get this we are liable to be that much more irritable.
- Diet: some people eat lots of sugar-rich food which sends their blood sugar level sky-high and then correspondingly low. Other people feed themselves so poorly that they are effectively suffering from malnutrition.
- Drugs: routinely consumed drugs such as caffeine, alcohol and nicotine are vastly underestimated in their effect. Recreational drugs can also devastate one's mood.
- Sleep: getting insufficient sleep on a regular basis is bad news indeed.

- Stress: having too much to do, too many pressures on you, tasks you find difficult to achieve, and other life stresses take a severe toll on your moods.
- Social factors: arguments with friends, relatives and workmates; bereavement, separation and divorce; simply feeling lonely – these are just some of the social factors that can affect your mood.

If you know that you sometimes get irritable, the chances are that there are several items on that list which look familiar to you. The good news is that we can work on them, and later on in Part Two of this book, we will see exactly what to do.

There are tremendous pay-offs here. Most people much prefer someone who is 'the same every day' to someone who is 'downright moody'.

Case study: Maya

Maya went through a period of three years in her late teens when, she said, she would 'snap anybody's head off who looked at me in the wrong way'. It turns out this wasn't quite true; there were just some days when she acted this way. Other days she was a thoroughly agreeable young person with lots of friends, a nice family life and occasional boyfriends. It turned out that the reason she was sometimes so irritable is that she was prone to getting quite depressed, mainly on account of her boyfriends being only 'occasional'. When she did feel depressed, however, she was snappy in the extreme, and even people's attempts to cheer her up provoked an abrasive reaction. Unsurprisingly, some of her friends drifted away, while even the ones that remained tended to treat her with some caution.

The solution to Maya's problems was twofold.

- First, she gradually worked on her depression until she settled in a fairly consistently happy mood. This was difficult, because she had set up a vicious circle whereby her depression caused her irritability, which caused some of her friends to desert her, which in turn exacerbated her depression. Nevertheless, she implemented three significant measures which helped her to be happier.
- Second, and while she was working on her depression, she also worked on the 'Response' box in our model. In other words, she trained herself to 'button my lip and count to ten' whenever she felt like snapping.

The net result is that both she and her friends feel that life is now more predictable and, partly as a result, more rewarding.

Summary

- Sometimes you may be more irritable than at other times. One day you may be in a good mood, the next in a bad mood. The key concept here is 'mood'.
- There are lots of factors that influence our mood, notably illness, routine, exercise, diet, drugs, sleep patterns, life stresses and social factors.
- We can work on these (as we shall see in Part Two) so that, if we want, we can be not only difficult to anger, but reliable and consistent: 'the same every day'!

9

What is the purpose of getting angry?

Rather like gravity, anger is part of life; so to start questioning whether it is good or bad is to head up a blind alley.
Perhaps we can do better by asking what purpose anger
serves. Most of the things that are 'part of the human condition' do serve a purpose and anger is no exception.

Possible purposes

One purpose may be to help to produce 'socialisation' in
other people: in other words, to encourage other people
to behave in the way we would like them to – or, more
accurately, to discourage other people from behaving in a
way we don't want them to. The distinction is not just a
question of semantics. It *is*, in fact, possible to influence
a person's behaviour much more by encouragement than
by punishment. This point was encapsulated by the old
cartoon depicting a fearsomely old-fashioned school with
a notice on the wall reading 'The beatings will continue
until morale improves', neatly making the point that some

things simply cannot be produced by beatings – or anger, or any other negative means. Nevertheless, for our present purposes it is worth noting that anger does indeed serve the purpose of discouraging behaviour that we don't want.

The trouble with this is that if we happen to be rather intolerant individuals, then we can feel there is a tremendous lot of 'behaviour we don't want', which in turn means that we will spend too much of our lives being angry.

On the other hand, if we ourselves are fairly tolerant individuals, and know what behaviour we like and dislike in each other, then anger can be a highly appropriate response, though of course in moderation. Maybe 'anger' is not really the right word in this context; possibly 'annoyance' is nearer the mark. If somebody cares for us and cares about what we think, then to see that their behaviour has annoyed us even slightly is sufficient to influence them.

One piece of good news is that there is much less undesirable behaviour than we think. Take the case of Tom and Emily, who were out for a day trip to the seaside with their children aged ten and twelve. It was 12.30 p.m., just coming up to lunchtime, when the family was walking past an ice-cream van near the beach. The ten-year-old asked for an ice cream, to which his father replied: 'No, it'll be lunchtime in a quarter of an hour.' The boy was not to be pacified, however, and persisted in trying to persuade and cajole his father into buying an ice cream, refusing even to move on past the van.

His father's response was to insist: 'If I say no, I mean no. If you really want one, then you can have one after lunch.'

This was no good; the ten-year-old wanted his ice cream there and then, and achieving this was evidently becoming more important than life itself. His father, for his part, felt that it was important to make a stand and show his son that you can't always have what you want.

Well, I will spare you the ghastly details, but suffice to say that that was the end of their day trip as any sort of enjoyable enterprise.

I talked to Tom about this afterwards in terms of the personality characteristics being displayed by the ten-year-old boy. What it boiled down to was that he was being very assertive and very persevering, both of which characteristics his father thought were admirable ones he'd want in his son when he became an adult. So, paradoxically, he felt he should be encouraging such characteristics rather than just getting angry when they are displayed!

This is only one small example of how tricky it can be to judge and appraise situations. Much more often than it seems at first sight, the characteristics that are being displayed when we are tempted to get annoyed are ones which, in other circumstances, we would value rather than condemn.

What it boils down to is that anger – or at least annoyance – can be entirely appropriate in order to express disapproval of other people's behaviour, *when we are really sure that we disapprove of it.*

Anger and motivation

Anger/annoyance also has another purpose, namely to

provide us with the motivation to do things we otherwise wouldn't do.

One of the angriest times I have ever experienced was when our nine-month-old daughter got locked in the car on a very hot summer's day, with the keys also in the car. Nearby was a man from the emergency rescue service who wouldn't help in spite of him being able to and our being members.

It was the middle of June, the baby was in her seat in the back of the car, and my wife had inadvertently locked the keys in the car. Distraught, she left the baby and the car and went on to the street, with our other daughter who was two, to seek help. As if the gods were really with her, she spotted a man wearing the uniform of the rescue service just fifty yards down the street. She explained her plight, to which the man replied: 'Are you a member?'

My wife said yes, she was, to which the reply was: 'Have you got your membership card?'

'Yes, it's in the car.'

And the man's response was: 'Well, I can't do anything without your membership card.'

However, in a fit of generosity he loaned her a coin to phone me up so that I could come with the spare keys. I got there as quickly as I could, gave my wife the spare keys and went to speak to the 'rescue' man.

I say 'speak to', but that is perhaps misrepresenting what followed. I gave him a full and thorough account of what I thought of him, lasting a good five minutes and much to the entertainment of some of the passers-by.

Now, if you had asked me one sunny June afternoon to go and advise a representative of a road rescue service on how he should behave if somebody has locked themselves out of – and their baby into – a car, I would probably have said that I had better things to do. It was only the rage I felt that fired me up to enthusiastically advise this particular man.

The same thing applies when we hear stories of people going to help strangers beaten up in the street, or countries declaring war on other countries that are trampling over the human rights of their neighbours.

How much anger is enough?

So, the interesting question arises as to how much anger we need to display in order to influence other people's behaviour. Clearly, there is a vast range available. As we said earlier, if a person cares about you and what you think, then your expression of even a hint of annoyance will probably be sufficient. If they don't care about you or what you think, then nothing you do will have much effect.

(In fact, different rules hold good for physically violent situations such as war. So, for the moment, let us confine ourselves to non-violent interpersonal situations.)

With anger, as with most other things, it is not a question of 'the more the better' if you want to be effective. The inverted U-curve, sometimes known as Aristotle's golden mean, holds good here. If you like graphs, this is the thing for you. It is normally drawn as shown in Figure 9.1. It suggests that a little bit of anger will have some effect; a bit more anger will have more effect; but if you increase the anger too much, then the effect comes down again.

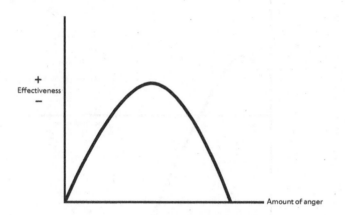

Figure 9.1 The traditional inverted U-curve

Actually, this 'traditional' inverted U is not quite what is needed in the case of anger. More accurate is the version shown in Figure 9.2. What this shows is that the 'best' amount of anger is just a small amount. If you increase it, the effectiveness decreases. And if you increase it even more, then the effectiveness is negative; in other words, what you are doing is counterproductive, and, far from influencing your target in the required direction, will provoke them to 'dig their heels in' or 'react against you'.

Effective Anger

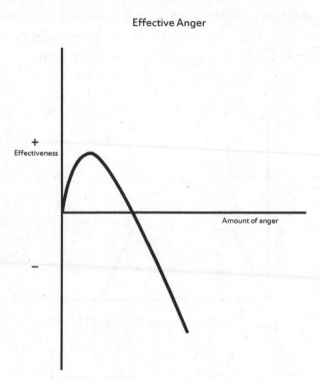

Figure 9.2 Graph showing effective anger

If you don't like graphs, forget this and think about someone who's not very good at making a cup of coffee. For the
sake of argument, let's agree that the best amount of coffee
to put in a mug is one rounded teaspoonful. So Lee comes
along, puts two rounded teaspoonfuls in his mug, adds boiling water and milk, sits down to enjoy it and finds it doesn't
taste very nice. Of course, he doesn't know *why* it doesn't
taste very nice because he's no good at making coffee. So

what does he do? He goes and puts in a third teaspoonful, which, of course, makes it taste even worse. And if he's really hopeless, he may even go back and add a fourth.

Now, the coffee example seems ridiculous to most of us because we know how much coffee to put in a mug. Not to Lee, though, because he's never made his own coffee before, and he has no idea how to do it. This is an exact parallel with some people and their anger. They start off by displaying too much anger and find that they don't get the desired result. So what do they do then? Get even angrier. To an onlooker this is as bizarre as Lee putting even more coffee in his mug when he already has too much. To the person concerned, however, it doesn't seem like that. 'If that much anger didn't work, then perhaps twice as much will,' they seem to be saying.

In summary, anger, like salt, is best in very small amounts, if at all. Too much ruins everything.

Does irritability have a purpose?

What about irritability? Does the same argument hold good there? The answer seems to be 'no', because the essence of irritability is that it is unjustified and inappropriate – more a reflection of your mood than of anything anybody else has done.

I have heard it said that the advantage of being known as 'irritable' is that it keeps everybody else 'on their toes'. The implication is that you will always be treated as carefully as though you were at your most irritable, because even when you are in a good mood people put it down to the fact that they are 'handling you with kid gloves'. So they carry on treating you that way.

For most people this has only a superficial attraction. Most people want to be respected and liked at work and in social situations, and liked and loved at home. While irritability may force others to *cover up* the manifestations of their disrespect and dislike for you, it does no more than that. There seems no shortcut to acquiring respect, liking and love, short of earning it. Being irritable normally means starting off with an overdraft.

Summary

- Anger is okay in the sense that most people get angry at some times; it's something we have to live with.
- Nevertheless, it does seem that we can influence the behaviour of those around us much more by positive means than becoming angry.
- Even so, anger – or at least annoyance – is a reasonable way of expressing displeasure of what somebody else does.
- In terms of how much anger is appropriate, it is almost always a lot less than we think. Indeed, too much anger is not only ineffective, it is actually counterproductive.

> • Irritability is never justified. After all, the fact that
>   it is unjustified is virtually part of its definition.

Exercise

Consider what you have read in this chapter, and answer
the following two questions to your satisfaction:

1. In general terms, not just for yourself, what purpose
   do you think anger most often serves?
2. For you specifically, what purpose do you think your
   anger most often serves?

PART TWO

SORTING IT OUT

Part Two of this book is all about solutions.

Having read Part One, you now know a lot about irritability and anger. However, knowing about a problem is not the same as solving that problem. So in this part of the book we examine all the possible solutions.

There are several ways of reading this part. Each chapter title gives you a pretty good idea of what is in the chapter and why you might want to read it. So you can, if you want, go straight to the chapters you think are most relevant to you and read those first. In fact, you will find it works even if you *just* read those, and omit the others. You can 'pick and choose'.

Alternatively, you can read steadily from here to the end, including every chapter whether or not it seems relevant at first sight. This isn't a bad idea, because some of the content may turn out to apply to you even though it might not have looked like it on first consideration. I have tried to include lots of examples, and some of them come up repeatedly; you might well find that you can easily identify with some of these cases.

At the end of each chapter is a summary and a project (or more than one!) to do. It is those projects which are really going to make a good impact for you if you follow them through.

Whichever way you tackle this part of the book, I hope you find it useful.

10

Getting a handle on the problem: the trigger

If you think back to Chapter 4, where we were starting to work on the model of irritability and anger, you may remember that the most basic model looked like Figure 10.1. This diagram doesn't contain the boxes we added as the model developed, but it does contain three of the most important ones. We can see that if any one of these three boxes is altered, then the whole sequence of irritability and anger comes to an end.

For example, take Justin, whose trigger is his neighbours playing music too loud. If that trigger doesn't happen, then the irritability and anger don't happen. Equally, even if the trigger does happen (the neighbours play their music), he still won't respond with anger if he appraises it as 'just them having a bit of fun – the thing to do is live and let live.' And finally, even if the trigger does happen and he appraises it as 'those awful people again – they need a good sorting out' he will still not display any irritability and anger if he takes himself off to see his friend in the adjoining road or puts his own headphones on.

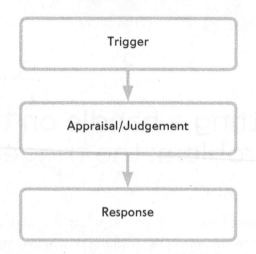

Figure 10.1 A model for analysing irritability and anger

So, this simple model yields three possible solutions:

1. somehow or other have the neighbours not play their music;
2. appraise it in a different light; or
3. respond in some different way.

In this particular example, which would you say is the best solution? Personally I'd go for either number 1 (ideally) or number 2.

Or what about Amy, who said she completely 'lost it' when she found her twelve-year-old daughter washing her hair in the bath instead of tidying her room? Again, there are three possible options:

1. She could have somehow got her daughter to tidy her room by a different means.
2. She could have appraised it a different way ('Well, at least she's keeping herself clean').
3. She could have responded in a different way, for example by taking herself off, calming down, and telling her daughter (again) that she expected her room to be tidied after she'd finished her bath.

Again it's a matter of personal opinion, but possibly numbers (2) or (3) would be the front-runners in this case:

And what about Omar, who gave a good roasting to the fifth guy who left the bar door open? In that case he could have:

1. Removed the trigger (by moving to a different table after the first couple of times).
2. Appraised it differently ('There are worse things in life than having to push a door closed every twenty minutes').
3. Responded differently, perhaps by asking each person to shut the door.

Possibly either (1) or (3) might be better in this case.

So, even with a simple three-box analysis some reasonably good solutions present themselves.

The odd thing is that in each of these cases the individual concerned had taken on a sort of 'victim role', as though they could do nothing about what was happening. So Justin blamed the neighbours ('What can you do if you've got neighbours like that?'), Amy told the story as just one more example of how 'difficult' her daughter was, and Omar saw his experience in the bar as one more example of how 'ignorant' (or ill-mannered) other people are.

Keeping a diary

In fact, there's no need to be a victim: there are lots of things we can do once we have 'got a handle on' the problem. In other words, *once you know, reliably, what triggers your anger or irritability you are halfway to sorting it out.* And if you want to know what triggers it, keeping a diary works very well.

The best form of diary to keep, in the first instance, is illustrated by Diary 1. You will see there are just two boxes: one for you to write about the trigger, and the other for you to write about how you responded. There is one blank copy of this diary included here, and there are more in the Appendix.

These diaries are very important. Their purpose is, as I've just said, to enable you to get a handle on what makes you irritable and angry. If you can do this, you are halfway home. So exactly how do you fill them in? The answer is: it is best to fill in a diary sheet each time you get irritable or angry, and to do it *as soon as possible* after the incident. It is also a good idea to make your accounts as complete as possible. On the following pages I have reproduced more or less what was filled in by several people we have already described, when they kept their diaries.

Diary 1

Keep a record of when you get irritable or angry. Fill it in as soon as possible after the event. Note as clearly as possible what triggered your irritability/anger, and how you responded.

Trigger (include day, date and time)

Response (what did you do?)

Example (a)

> **Trigger** (include day, date and time)
>
> Saturday 3 June, 11.15 a.m. The kids next door were playing soccer in the street outside. They had already been across the lawn several times and finally the ball hit our front window.

> **Response** (what did you do?)
>
> I went straight out, took the ball off the kids, rang the bell next door and gave their mother a piece of my mind.

Example (b)

> **Trigger** (include day, date and time)
>
> Tuesday 3 June, 8.00 p.m. We were sitting, eating a meal when, yet again, my husband was chewing his food so loudly that half the street would be able to hear him. I'm sure he does it just to annoy me, or at least he doesn't care that it does annoy me. What he does is to get his mouth full of food and then spend ages chewing every mouthful and talking to me while he does it.

Response (what did you do?)

I didn't say or do anything, I just felt really tight inside. And I didn't talk to him properly and I just felt sad being married to him. I've told him about it dozens of times before, so what's the point going on about it again? But somehow it just symbolises the way he is – he doesn't care about me, just about him.

Example (c)

Trigger (include day, date and time)

Wednesday 7 June, 3.30 p.m. The boss asked me to go out to Scudamore Avenue to sort out a call there. The occupier wanted some wiring looked at that they weren't sure was safe. The thing is that the boss knew I already had plenty of work on and he was just taking advantage of me because he knew I wouldn't complain.

Response (what did you do?)

I was just very short with him so that he would know I was irritated and thought he was out of order. But I finished off the work that had to be done in the base and then went off and sorted this other person's wiring out. And I did the jobs properly.

Example (d)

Trigger (include day, date and time)

Thursday 10 April, 6.30 p.m. I had been on at my daughter all day long to tidy her room and she kept saying she would do it in a minute, or a bit later. Then at about half past six I found her sitting in the bath just washing her hair – and deliberately provoking me, saying, 'What are you going to do about that, then?'

Response (what did you do?)

I really let rip. I shouted and screamed at her for – it must have been ten minutes. She went really pale, and looking back at it I was over the top. But it worked, she did tidy her room later on.

Example (e)

Trigger (include day, date and time)

Wednesday 27 July, 4.15 p.m. There was no real trigger beyond the fact that I was feeling very stressed out, as usual. At work these days there are just so many demands on me from so many different people that I cannot possibly fulfil everything that everybody expects of me. Therefore, when Jason just made some throwaway remark, that was the last straw.

Response (what did you do?)

I just blew my top at Jason and criticised him for his attitude. It was totally unfair, what he had said was just by way of banter. Me blowing my top was much more to do with my state of mind than Jason's attitude. But anyway I apologised to him later on and things seem to be okay now, more or less.

Reading your diary

Well, never mind reading your diary for the moment. Let's first of all get good at reading other people's diaries.

Even before that, let's recap on what the point of reading these diaries is: it is *to obtain insight into what makes you irritable and angry, so that you can take action about it.* And, to do that, you will first of all have to develop the skill of reading diaries astutely.

Now let's take the examples in order.

First of all, look again at the example in which Marius tells how he was driven to distraction by his neighbour's kids playing football in the street. Which of the following possibilities do you think was the trigger:

1. The kids repeatedly running across his grass.
2. The ball hitting his window.

3. The thought that his neighbours showed no consideration for him.
4. The belief that kids playing in the street makes the area look poor?

In this particular case the answer Marius gave was both (1) and (2); but what really irritated Marius was that the neighbours had no consideration for people around them, and indeed made the street look like a rough area. So in a way Marius's anger had more to do with his appraisal and judgement of the trigger, rather than the trigger itself. Nevertheless, if he wants to sort out his irritability and anger he needs to spot the 'visible' trigger of the boys playing soccer. Once he knows this is his weak spot, then he can sort out how to reappraise it, if that is what he decides on. If Marius wanted to become less irritated and angry, he could view the children playing outside in a different light. He could view it simply as 'kids having a good time' and 'showing that the street is a lively place to live'. Do you think that is likely to work with this man? No, neither did I.

So what is left? In this case, the main thing is to look in the response box. His response was to take the ball from the kids and storm round and shout at their mother. What other response do you think he might have made? Which of the following do you think would be best:

1. Switch on the television, turn the volume up loud until their game is over.
2. Every time the kids appear on the street, go round to

their mother and put his point of view in as friendly a way as possible.

3. Do nothing, just blank it all from his mind?
4. To take 'opposite action' (as American psychologist Marsha Linehan refers to it). This means, for example in this case, to go out onto the street and join in the game of soccer. Not to make some kind of convoluted point, but genuinely enjoying a game of football with the boys every time they go out.

Which would you go for? I would suggest that option (2) is good: to go round and put his point of view, amicably, just as often as he likes, just as soon as the kids appear on the street. Option (4) is good too though, and might transform the situation – he might find himself genuinely enjoying things, depending on whether he can persuade himself to do so, and maybe improve his ball skills as well!

Many angry and irritable people make the mistake of thinking that the best reaction is (3), to 'do nothing at all'. This is not necessarily the case. It may be right to stick up for your rights, assertively. But 'assertive' does not mean 'angry' or 'aggressive'. Or maybe it's best to stick up for your emotional wellbeing, in which case option 4 would suit some people best.

So, in this example perhaps the best bet is for Marius to alter his response; and this is what he did. Nevertheless, the starting point was for him to be clear about what triggered his anger, rather than just thinking he was generally bad-tempered.

What about the case of Aisha, who is so acutely annoyed by her husband when he eats noisily. Again, what do you think was the 'real' trigger for her annoyance:

1. The sheer decibel-level of her husband's eating – he should learn to eat more quietly.
2. The fact that he carried on talking to her while he was still chewing.
3. The fact that she saw it as symbolising their incompatibility.
4. The fact that she had nothing better to do than worry about how much noise her husband made when he was eating?

Numbers (1) and (2) are the literal triggers. So how could we remove them? Earplugs to cut down the decibel-level won't help. Talk to him while he is chewing so that he isn't tempted to talk while chewing? Perhaps not.

Really, the problem lies in Aisha's appraisal that the chewing symbolises their incompatibility. So, ultimately, it is either that – or their incompatibility itself – that needs working on. Nevertheless, she does need to be clear on the initial trigger so that she can take action on it. In the interim she might also ask him to chew a bit more quietly. But that would probably be missing the point.

Another example involved Lola's teenage son Nathaniel, who dropped a mug on the floor and broke it. Again, what was the trigger:

1. The mug breaking.
2. The cost of the mug.
3. The loud noise the mug made when it hit the floor.
4. Lola's appraisal that Nathaniel is careless and needs to be taught a lesson?

Well, number (1) is obviously the 'literal' answer, but it is quickly followed by number (4). Clearly, once Lola knows what the triggers are for her thinking like that ('he is careless and needs to be taught a lesson') she can prepare a more helpful appraisal and train herself to use it at such times. (Such an appraisal might be: 'We all drop things on the floor from time to time, youngsters especially. There's no need to get uptight about it.')

So, what have we got so far, from looking at these first examples?

- It is sometimes quite difficult to see exactly what the trigger is, because the 'literal' trigger and the appraisal are jumbled together.
- It is worthwhile disentangling these two aspects, because then you can prepare a more helpful appraisal if need be, and be ready to use it next time the trigger for your irritation and anger appears.
- Keeping a diary, on the model of Diary 1, is helpful in doing this.

> • Often the key lies in learning a different response, for example tackling the neighbour in a different way, asking people to shut the door, tackling the underlying issue of compatibility, telling the youngster to brush up the broken mug. But the same argument applies; before we can prepare a more helpful response, we need to be clear about what triggers our irritation and anger.

Let's move on now and have a look at the other examples. Let's consider Brandon, the electrician who was asked to do too much by his boss. What was the real trigger:

1. Being overloaded with work.
2. Feeling he is being put-upon by his boss?

Clearly the literal trigger is being overloaded with work. Feeling put-upon by his boss is the appraisal Brandon makes.

There is another example, to do with a stressed-out executive, Nish, of whom I will tell you more later. He described the trigger for one occasion of large-scale irritability as:

1. Trying to cope with more work than he could reasonably do.
2. A colleague being tactless.
3. Just being in a bad mood that day.

From his account it sounds as though it was a combination of all three. Certainly he was overloaded with work, so he was in 'a bad mood'; but also perhaps the colleague was a shade tactless. Triggers can sometimes be slightly complex, as in 'my colleague being tactless when I'm overworked and in a bad mood'. Quite possibly none of the three elements mentioned (tactlessness, overwork, bad mood) would cause him to be irritable *on its own*.

Reading your diary (again)

The previous section will have got you pretty good at reading diaries in general – which means that you are also going to be pretty good at reading your own.

So all you have to do now is keep a diary of most of the times you get irritable and angry, along the lines described. Then analyse it to determine your triggers.

What you are looking for is a (short) list of triggers for your irritation and anger. Here are some that other people have produced:

- the neighbours playing loud music
- the kids next door playing soccer in the street
- the people next door showing no consideration for their neighbours
- other people being inconsiderate (as in the bar door)

- other people putting themselves above me (as in queue-jumping)
- my husband eating his food noisily
- my husband/wife
- my children
- my partner
- George, at work
- my son being careless
- being kept waiting
- being contradicted or proved wrong in public
- being overworked by my boss
- being dumped by my boyfriend
- my partner telling other people about things which were just between us
- my wife laughing and joking with other men
- being made to look foolish in public
- my daughter being lazy
- my daughter being disobedient
- my son telling lies
- people stealing from me or damaging my property
- bouncers
- police officers
- being hungry
- being carved up by another driver
- being crammed in the Tube
- being stressed out
- being bored
- being tired

Summary

- It is important to have a very clear idea of what triggers your irritation and anger.

- Once you have that, you can either remove the trigger (although this is frequently impossible) or take a range of other actions, which we will cover later on.

- The best way of identifying what triggers your irritation and anger is to keep a diary; simply trying to recollect what triggers it is surprisingly unreliable. A good diary form for you to use (Diary 1) is included here and in the Appendix.

- When you keep your diary you will find that you sometimes confuse triggers with appraisals (for example, writing the trigger down as 'half a dozen selfish so-and-so's down the bar' rather than 'half a dozen people coming in and leaving the door open'). Nevertheless, this can be helpful because, once you come to make your final (short) list of what triggers your anger, you may decide that the 'real' trigger is indeed 'other people's selfishness' rather than 'doors being left open'.

- A list of the triggers that other people have found for their anger is given on pages 123–24; this may be helpful as a starting point when compiling your own.

Project

- Probably by keeping the diary (Diary 1), get a crystal clear idea of what triggers your irritation and anger. It may be specific (people leaving the lounge door open) or diffuse (my son being careless — which could be manifested in lots of ways), external (someone else doing something, e.g. dropping a mug on the floor) or internal (within you, e.g. being bored, being tired). However you do it, become an absolute expert on what makes you irritable or angry, so that if someone were to ask, you could give them a vivid description of what does it for you.

- If possible, remove those triggers. You will find that this is surprisingly difficult. Some triggers can be removed, others cannot. Don't worry in either case. The following chapters will show you what to do if the trigger can't be removed. Nevertheless, if you can easily get rid of it, do so.

- Tip: some people see 'getting rid of the trigger' as 'cheating' — they feel they should learn to deal with the trigger. I disagree; if you can get rid of something that makes you angry then to me it seems plain common sense to do so. Having said that, we will also look at how to deal with the trigger.

11

Why do I get angry? 1: appraisal/judgement

What you will learn in this chapter

- The answer to the question posed in the chapter title: to put it more fully: 'Why do I always get irritated and angry at things that don't bother other people, and how do I sort it out?'
- The most common errors made in the appraisals and judgements people make of triggering situations.
- How to analyse some of the examples we have covered so far in terms of those common errors, so you get good at identifying such errors.
- How to make better appraisals and judgements and avoid the errors described.
- How to change your own behaviour – permanently.

Why do I always get irritated and angry at things that don't bother other people?

We covered this earlier on, but just by way of revision:

- A potential trigger for anger occurs: e.g. you find your twelve-year-old daughter in the bath washing her hair instead of tidying her room, having been asked to do so repeatedly.
- You make an appraisal/judgement of that situation which is likely to produce anger: e.g. 'She's deliberately being defiant, she's just trying to wind me up.' (It's worth noting at this stage that there is a possible alternative appraisal along the lines of 'Well, she's not tidying her room but at least she's keeping herself clean and tidy.')
- Assuming you made the anger-inducing appraisal, anger ensues.
- Your inhibitions may be strong enough to prevent the anger becoming apparent to anybody else.
- Or possibly your inhibitions are not that strong, so the potential recipient gets a piece of your mind: e.g. the daughter gets shouted at.

In Part One we summarised this process with the model shown again here in Figure 11.1.

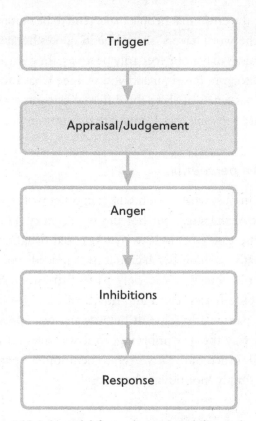

Figure 11.1 A model for analysing irritability and anger

Appraising and judging in triggering situations: the most common thinking errors

Psychiatrist and psychotherapist Aaron T Beck completed a great deal of research into the kind of thinking errors that people make. And it turns out that such errors are not random: the errors that people make tend to be quite specific. Maybe the word 'errors' should be in quotes because while the appraisals may not necessarily be *wrong*, they are generally *unhelpful* to you. Read on and you will see what I mean.

Beck has given labels to the different categories of errors. Below are the ones that I think are the most important.

Selective perception

This means just what it sounds like: in other words, a person sees part of the story but not the whole story. For example, in the case of Amy's twelve-year-old daughter sitting in the bath washing her hair, she was indeed 'not tidying her room' – but that was only part of the story. She was also keeping herself clean and tidy. In fact, as it turns out, this was particularly relevant because she was appearing in a school play the next morning, so it was relevant that she was 'well turned out'. However, to her mother's perception she was simply 'not tidying her room'.

Mind-reading

Again, this is exactly what it says. In our example it is manifested by Amy saying: 'She does it deliberately to wind me up.' How does she know her daughter does it to wind her up? The only possible answer can be by mind-reading. The point is that mind-reading is impossible, as far as we know. Amy has no idea whether her daughter is really trying to wind her up deliberately or not, so it is unhelpful to jump to that conclusion. She might just as well jump to the opposite conclusion, that her daughter is *not* trying to wind her up deliberately. This is a very common way of thinking: many people assume that the person who irritates them does it deliberately.

All or nothing thinking

This is where, when we don't get what we want, we will see the situation as 'awful'. So, to take this example again, whereas some mothers, having failed to get their daughters to tidy their rooms, would tell somebody else: 'I wish I could get my daughter to tidy her room. Do you know I spent all day nagging her to do it yesterday and still she didn't do it', other mothers will see it as 'awful' and 'the end of the world'. It is an example of 'all or nothing thinking': seeing things as *either* wonderful *or* terrible, *either* perfect *or* awful, etc. It is good practice to develop the habit of thinking and talking in shades of grey, where, for example, events may be 'not as I want' but are not necessarily 'awful'.

Use of emotive language

Which is the particularly emotive word that Amy used about her twelve-year-old daughter? The one that I would pick out is 'defiant'. She viewed her daughter as being deliberately defiant. This is a very strong word designed to make adversaries of mother and daughter. If one person defies another, then surely it is the first person's duty to overcome that defiance. This is likely to be a very unhelpful way of phrasing things.

Incidentally, although I am writing this as though we are talking out loud to somebody else, when we make our judgements the 'conversation' is with ourselves, so the language is even more emotive. We can think nothing of referring to other people, even our own family, using words we may never use out loud about anybody to anybody!

Overgeneralisation

This is where we notice a particular observation that is true (e.g. that the girl in question has not tidied her room) and then make a sweeping generalisation from that fact (e.g. 'She's bone idle' or 'She never does anything I ask her to'). It is usually far better to stick to the accurate statement, i.e. 'It is difficult to get her to tidy her room.' This of course puts her on a par with just about every other youngster, and it also clarifies what the problem is (trying to get her to tidy her room). Overgeneralisations are very common and usually very destructive.

Project

These five types of thinking errors in appraisal and judgement are very important. Therefore I would like you to stop reading for a moment and just look back over the five headings; then see if you can think of an example for each of the five where you have actually thought or reacted in the way described. In other words:

- An example of you showing selective perception (noticing only one aspect of a situation).
- An example of where you were 'mind-reading' (assuming you knew someone's intention when you could not possibly have done so).
- An example of 'all or nothing thinking' (where you portrayed to yourself that what has happened is absolutely 'awful' rather than just 'not what you would have wished').
- An example of you using emotive language to yourself (describing an event in a way which is almost bound to get you 'fired up').
- An example of you 'overgeneralising' (noticing something that is true, but going way over the top with a generalisation of it).

However, take care not to blame yourself for any of these; all of them are very common indeed, but are usually unhelpful for you.

What thinking errors are being made in these appraisals/judgements?

Below are a number of examples of triggers, along with the appraisal/judgement that was made by the recipient. After each example is a list of the five thinking errors people may typically make in their appraisals/judgements. Your task is to <u>underline</u> all the errors which apply to each example (sadly, one appraisal can exhibit several of the errors). You may wish to circle the error which you think is the main one in each case.

The first three examples have been done for you:

1. *Trigger:* Justin has noisy neighbours playing music loudly next door. This happens every week or so and normally lasts for an hour or two.

   Justin's appraisal: 'They do that deliberately to annoy me – they don't give a damn about what I think.'

   Error(s): selective perception / <u>mind-reading</u> / all or nothing thinking / <u>emotive language</u> / overgeneralising.

2. *Trigger:* Marius's neighbours' kids are playing football in the street outside. This happens every few days and normally their game lasts for about forty-five minutes.

   Marius's appraisal: 'They're a bloody nuisance, they've got no respect for anybody, it makes it not worth living here.'

Error(s): selective perception / mind-reading / all or nothing thinking / <u>emotive language</u> / <u>overgeneralising</u>.

3. *Trigger:* A fifth man comes into the bar where Omar is sitting with Carlos and Ryan and leaves a door open (four others having done so previously).

   Omar's appraisal: 'They just don't give a damn about anybody.'

   Error(s): selective perception / <u>mind-reading</u> / all or nothing thinking / <u>emotive language</u> / <u>overgeneralising</u>.

4. *Trigger:* Aisha's husband eats food noisily and talks to her at the same time.

   Aisha's appraisal: 'I just can't stand the way he eats, it just shows how he's not my type of person.'

   Error(s): selective perception / mind-reading / all or nothing thinking / emotive language / overgeneralising.

5. *Trigger:* Lola's teenage son Nathaniel drops a china mug on the floor and it breaks. (Note: we know that Nathaniel takes great care over his homework.)

   Lola's appraisal: 'He doesn't take any care about anything, he just doesn't give a damn.'

   Error(s): selective perception / mind-reading / all or nothing thinking / emotive language / overgeneralising.

6. *Trigger:* Nicole has to wait a long time in the outpatient department with her five-year-old daughter. Having witnessed the doctor and nurse working carefully with a number of patients, she then sees them having a tea-break after an hour and a half, relaxing and chatting to each other.

   Nicole's appraisal: 'They don't care about any of us, all they are interested in doing is relaxing and flirting with each other.'

   Error(s): selective perception / mind-reading / all or nothing thinking / emotive language / overgeneralising.

7. *Trigger:* Out at a party, Errol's wife contradicts him several times in front of others.

   Errol's appraisal: 'She's doing it deliberately to show me up and make me look small – I just can't stand her any longer.'

   Error(s): selective perception / mind-reading / all or nothing thinking / emotive language / overgeneralising.

8. *Trigger:* Brandon's otherwise fair boss asks him to do another task towards the end of the day which will take him over his normal finishing time.

   Brandon's appraisal: 'He always treats me unfairly, he's just a lousy bastard.'

   Error(s): selective perception / mind-reading / all or nothing thinking / emotive language / overgeneralising.

9.   *Trigger:* Danny has told his long-time partner Vicky something he took to be in confidence. Vicky, however, has told several other people about this.

     Danny's appraisal: 'That's totally out of order – she has got absolutely no sense of what's right and wrong.'

     Error(s): selective perception / mind-reading / all or nothing thinking / emotive language / overgeneralising.

10. *Trigger:* Lemy and Ella have been married several years. Ella has never had an extra-marital relationship and is generally a very good partner for Lemy. However, she does sometimes laugh and joke with other men.

     Lemy's appraisal: 'She's got no loyalty whatsoever; if I turned my back on her she'd be off like a shot.'

     Error(s): selective perception / mind-reading / all or nothing thinking / emotive language / overgeneralising.

The answers I would give are as follows:

4.   *Trigger:* Aisha's husband eats food noisily and talks to her at the same time.

     Aisha's appraisal: 'I just can't stand the way he eats, it just shows how he's not my type of person.'

     Error(s): selective perception / mind-reading / all or nothing thinking / <u>emotive language</u> / <u>overgeneralising</u>.

5. *Trigger:* Lola's teenage son Nathaniel drops a china mug on the floor and it breaks. (Note: we know that Nathaniel takes great care over his homework.)

    Lola's appraisal: 'He doesn't take any care about anything, he just doesn't give a damn.'

    Error(s): <u>selective perception</u> / mind-reading / all or nothing thinking / <u>emotive language</u> / overgeneralising.

6. *Trigger:* Nicole has to wait a long time in the outpatient department with her five-year-old daughter. Having witnessed the doctor and nurse working carefully with a number of patients, she then sees them having a tea-break after an hour and a half, relaxing and chatting to each other.

    Nicole's appraisal: 'They don't care about any of us, all they are interested in doing is relaxing and flirting with each other.'

    Error(s): <u>selective perception</u> / <u>mind-reading</u> / all or nothing thinking / emotive language / overgeneralising.

7. *Trigger:* Out at a party, Errol's wife contradicts him several times in front of others.

    Errol's appraisal: 'She's doing it deliberately to show me up and make me look small – I just can't stand her any longer.'

    Error(s): selective perception / <u>mind-reading</u> / all or nothing thinking / emotive language / <u>overgeneralising</u>.

8. *Trigger:* Brandon's otherwise fair boss asks him to do another task towards the end of the day which will take him over his normal finishing time.

   Brandon's appraisal: 'He always treats me unfairly, he's just a lousy bastard.'

   Error(s): <u>selective perception</u> / mind-reading / all or nothing thinking / <u>emotive language</u> / <u>overgeneralising</u>.

9. *Trigger:* Danny has told his long-time partner Vicky something he took to be in confidence. Vicky, however, has told several other people about this.

   Danny's appraisal: 'That's totally out of order – she has got absolutely no sense of what's right and wrong.'

   Error(s): <u>selective perception</u> / mind-reading / all or nothing thinking / emotive language / <u>overgeneralising</u>.

10. *Trigger:* Lemy and Ella have been married several years. Ella has never had an extra-marital relationship and is generally a very good partner for Lemy. However, she does sometimes laugh and joke with other men.

    Lemy's appraisal: 'She's got no loyalty whatsoever; if I turned my back on her she'd be off like a shot.'

    Error(s): <u>selective perception</u> / <u>mind-reading</u> / all or nothing thinking / emotive language / overgeneralising.

Summary of the main appraisal/judgement errors

- Selective perception: Where one or more important aspects of the situation are unnoticed.
- Mind-reading: Where a person believes s/he knows what is in another person's mind, especially their intention.
- All or nothing thinking: Where some unwanted event is viewed as awful, tragic, terrible, disastrous, etc., rather than simply unwelcome.
- Emotive language: Using strong language to oneself, almost automatically producing an angry reaction.
- Overgeneralisation: Making a sweeping generalisation from one true observation.

12

Working on your thinking

Applying the work on appraisals and judgments – and the thinking errors we can make – to your own situation

Now you've shown you can analyse other examples, you need some examples from your own life to work on. To get these, we need a slightly more sophisticated diary, as shown overleaf.

Diary 2

Fill this in as soon as possible after each time you get irritable or angry.

Trigger: Describe here what a video camera would have seen or heard. Include the day and date, but do not put what you thought or how you reacted.

_____

_____

_____

_____

Appraisal/Judgement: Write here the thoughts that went through your mind, as clearly as you can remember them.

_____

_____

_____

_____

Anger: Leave this blank for the time being.

_____

_____

_____

_____

Inhibitions: Leave this blank for the time being.

_____

_____

_____

_____

Response: Write here what a video camera would have seen you do and heard you say, as clearly as you can.

_____

_____

_____

_____

More helpful appraisal/judgement: How else might you have appraised the situation? To determine this, you might like to consider the following: What errors are you making (selective perception, mind-reading, all or nothing thinking, emotive language, overgeneralisation)?

_____

_____

_____

_____

If you had an all-knowing, all-wise friend, how would s/he have seen the situation?

Is a reframing of the situation possible? (A glass that is half empty is also half full.)

What would your cost–benefit analysis be of seeing the situation the way you did?

_____

_____

_____

_____

Methods of making your appraisals/ judgements more helpful

There are four major ways of doing this.

Identify and remove 'thinking errors'

This starts with analysing your appraisal/judgement. So, for example, Amy, who saw her daughter 'not tidying her room', might realise that this was selective perception. In other words, while it was true the girl was not tidying her room, she was washing her hair and thereby making herself clean and tidy for the next morning's school play. This positive aspect of the girl's behaviour was something that had completely eluded Amy. She had truly only perceived the fact that her daughter was not tidying her room. Once this 'error' had been spotted, the situation almost automatically rectified itself.

In the same way, Amy might also see that she was 'mind-reading', another 'error'. In this instance she was saying to herself that her daughter was 'deliberately winding her up'. Clearly this is mind-reading; how could the mother possibly know that the daughter had that intention? Once this has been spotted as an 'error', Amy believed it less firmly.

She also recognised that she was 'awfulising'. In other words, she was making the fact that her daughter had not tidied her room into the 'biggest thing in the world' – in her own words, 'getting it out of proportion'.

She was also using emotive language, describing her daughter as 'defiant'. This is a strong word which produces strong emotional reactions. What is more, it is also mind-reading: it implies that Amy can tell that the daughter has a particular motive in mind. The 'error' of using emotive language is easily corrected – you simply refrain from using it. You simply delete from your mind the phrase where the word 'defiant' was used.

And the final error is overgeneralisation: in this instance, saying that the daughter was 'bone idle'. This was not actually true: there are all sorts of other things that the daughter did perfectly well (for example, keeping herself clean and tidy, joining in the school play, etc.). Again, in this instance once the 'error' has been spotted, the situation almost automatically corrects itself.

It is perhaps worth making the point that there are very few examples generally that illustrate all five errors simultaneously, and that is why this episode of Amy and her daughter is something of a 'collectors' item'!

The 'friend technique'

This is where you say to yourself: If I had an all-knowing, all-wise friend, someone who had only my interests at heart, how would s/he appraise this situation so that it worked out best for me?

In this instance the friend might say something like 'Come on, Amy, just leave the girl alone. She's a good girl, and at least she's keeping herself clean and tidy, which is a step ahead of a lot of kids. Anyway, how many kids do you know who tidy their rooms when their mums ask them to?'

This can be a powerful technique if you practice it regularly and if you can build up a good image of this all-knowing, all-wise friend. It does not have to be anybody real – perhaps it's helpful if it isn't – just so long as it is a very wise person who has your interests at heart, someone who is always on your side.

Incidentally, some people prefer to do it the other way around: in other words, ask themselves: 'What would you say to a friend in this situation, a really good friend to whom you wanted to offer constructive support?'

Reframing the trigger

Most 'bad news' can also be reframed as 'good news'. The most famous example is the glass of water that is half empty (bad news). It is of course also half full (good news).

So how might you reframe the situation where, in spite of being nagged all day long, your twelve-year-old daughter is sitting in the bath washing her hair rather than tidying her room? There are in fact several options here. One is to simply focus on the good aspect, the 'half full' aspect: namely, in this case, the fact that she is keeping herself clean and tidy and preparing for the school play. Another is that clearly the daughter feels relaxed enough with her mother, and 'un-frightened' enough of her, not to feel that she has to do exactly what she's told. This 'quality of relationship' aspect is normally viewed as good news and would not usually produce anger. A third possible reframe is that in fact the daughter is displaying assertiveness and perseverance by not simply doing what she is told. Both these characteristics are rightly viewed as good qualities to encourage in youngsters.

Some situations are much more difficult to reframe. Take the example of Omar, where every other person who comes into the bar leaves the door open: how might that be reframed? It is very difficult to see anything intrinsically good about people leaving the door open just near where you are sitting. On the other hand, if you look at the situation from a much wider perspective, maybe it is just possible. The overall situation is, after all, that there you are sitting with two friends having a good drink and a talk and occasionally somebody leaves the door open. Supposing you were to have a conversation with someone who had just lost all he owned in an earthquake in Turkey, or a man who had lost his loved ones in the floods in Bangladesh, or a woman who had lost everything and everybody in a natural catastrophe in South America. Suppose you were to suggest to this individual that there is a man sitting in a bar drinking happily with his two friends who views it as a disaster when several people leave the door by him open. What sort of reaction would you be likely to get?

That, strictly speaking, is reframing: it puts the event in a different context. And it might just sway the person concerned; you might just be able to use it. Curiously, though, my experience is that it *doesn't* often do the trick. Only when there is real personal relevance (as in the first example of seeing the twelve-year-old daughter as 'a good kid looking after herself and getting ready for the play at school next day') do people really latch onto it. Nevertheless, I mentioned the second example of reframing because it is one that works well for me personally; so, who knows, it might work for you too.

Cost–benefit analysis

Doing a cost–benefit analysis of your appraisal/judgement is, happily, not half so difficult as it sounds. It's really just a matter of looking at the pros and cons.

For consistency's sake it would probably be a good idea to stick to just one example for the most part while we go through these options, namely our mother Amy with her twelve-year-old daughter. But I'm getting a bit fed up with that example, so let's look instead at Aaron, a father with a son, also aged twelve, who hadn't done his homework properly but said he had so he could watch television.

When Aaron had a look at the homework and saw how little had been done his appraisal was something like this: 'The boy's a liar, he's tried to pull the wool over my eyes, where's he going to get to in life if he carries on like this? He'll come to no good, all the other kids at school will do better than him . . .'

Clearly this is a piece of selective perception in that there are probably other aspects to the boy that we haven't been told about; his life cannot begin and end with that one piece of undone homework. Nevertheless, the father's appraisal/ judgement may indeed turn out to be correct. The only thing is, we would have to wait for a number of years before we would find out one way or the other. And even then it might only be correct because it was a self-fulfilling prophecy.

In the meantime, what are the pros and cons of making an appraisal/judgement like that? Let's do the cons (against) first:

- It agitates the father.
- It makes the boy feel inadequate.
- It worsens the relationship between father and son.
- It labels school work as a thoroughly punishing business that no boy in his right mind would ever want to do.

. . . and there are probably more cons that you can think of. On the 'pro' side there's – well, very little that I can see. Possibly it might motivate the son to do more homework next time; but then again, it might motivate him to be a bit more devious next time so he can get away with it.

What about an appraisal/judgement along the lines of: 'The kid has clearly got no idea what he's doing, I'd better see if I can help him out or see if he knows somebody else who can if I can't'? Clearly the cost–benefit analysis in this case swings right round the other way. The benefits of such an appraisal are:

- An improvement in the father–son relationship.
- Better school work.
- Probably more openness about how things are going . . .

. . . and so on. The costs are probably significant too: predominantly, a drain on the father's time. On balance, however, the second appraisal/judgement produces a much better cost–benefit analysis for all concerned than the first one.

Now, you may say that you can't decide how to think on the basis of a cost–benefit analysis; you think according to what is 'true'. Well, maybe; but I'm not convinced, because we've seen that it is very difficult to see what is 'true' in this instance – and indeed in many others. And moreover, if you look at how people do think, even down to something as tangible as which political party to vote for, it very often is to do with what would benefit them the most and cost them the least.

The main methods of producing more helpful appraisals/judgements

- Identify the error (selective perception, mind-reading, all or nothing thinking, emotive language or overgeneralisation) and correct it.
- The 'friend technique'. How would an all-knowing, all-wise friend advise you to view the situation?
- Reframe the situation. Search for the good aspects of it, or, failing that, view it from a completely different perspective.
- Conduct a cost–benefit analysis. That is, examine the costs and benefits of appraising the situation the way you are, and then look for a more cost-effective way.

Exercise

Lemy's wife, Ella, likes to laugh and joke with other men – merely in high spirits, with no intention of getting involved in an extra-marital relationship. Lemy, however, gets jealous and produces an appraisal/judgement along the lines of: 'She's showing me up, people will think I'm not making her happy, I'm losing face, she's out of order.'

1. What alternative appraisal would an all-knowing, all-wise friend make?
2. How might Lemy reframe this behaviour?
3. What would a cost–benefit analysis of Lemy's appraisal look like? Can you suggest a better appraisal?

Below are the kind of answers that I produced, but I would suggest that you produce your own before you have a look at these:

1. A reassuring friend might say, 'Come on, Lemy, you know perfectly well that Ella is as faithful as the day is long, she'd never let you down, she thinks you're the best thing since sliced bread. She just likes to have lots of fun but everybody knows what she thinks of you.'

2. Lemy might reframe the situation as: 'It's good that Ella feels secure enough in our relationship that she can have a great time and know that I won't take it amiss and neither would anybody else.'

3. A cost–benefit analysis of Lemy's original appraisal/judgement is that the 'costs' are rather heavy: his appraisal will make him anxious, jealous and possibly angry. It will put a strain on the relationship, it will limit Ella's activities, make her feel that Lemy doesn't trust her and generally put a dampener on all their activities. The only benefit of such an appraisal is that at least it lets Ella know that Lemy cares about her – but she probably knows that anyway. Yes, a better appraisal would be along the lines of (1) or (2) above.

Let's look at another example . . .

Exercise

Vicky, while being interviewed on a radio programme, mentioned that her husband Danny likes to wear her thongs. Danny, who is also in the public eye, took a very dim view of this, making an appraisal/judgement along the lines of: 'Has she got no sense? Doesn't she realise that some things are just between us? Is she deliberately trying to make my life as difficult as possible? She's just completely stupid!' Needless to say, this made Danny very angry with Vicky.

1. What error of thinking was Danny making
2. What alternative appraisal would an all-knowing, all-wise friend make?
3. How might Danny reframe what Vicky did?
4. What would a cost–benefit analysis of Danny's appraisal look like? Can you suggest a better appraisal?

Again, there is a list of answers that I would make below, but I would suggest that you produce your own before you have a look at these.

1. Danny is making a lot of thinking errors. Particularly, he is using emotive language ('she's completely stupid') and overgeneralising (just because she has said one thing – or even several things – which would be best left unsaid, it does not mean that she is completely stupid; probably there are lots of other things which would suggest she is far from stupid). One might also say that Danny is mind-reading (assuming that

Vicky is trying to make his life as difficult as possible). Likewise, you could say that he is indulging in selective perception (because Vicky probably does other things which make his life good) and you might even say he is thinking in all or nothing terms (is it really so bad that people know that he and his wife have an intimate side to their relationship?).

2. An all-knowing, all-wise friend might say, 'Come on Danny, there's no need to make quite such a big deal out of it. You know that Vicky thinks the world of you and wouldn't deliberately do things to make things difficult for you. So what if other people rib you a bit? It only shows that they're jealous. Just put it to one side.'

3. How might Danny reframe what Vicky said and did? He might say that it is good that Vicky feels so relaxed and secure in their relationship that she doesn't have to watch every word she says, even when she's being interviewed on nation-wide radio. He might even say that it adds to his street-cred that he has a pretty adventurous private life as well as the public one that most people see. He could even relish the fact that other people are made envious by what she said.

4. A cost–benefit analysis would look something like this. The costs of the appraisal that Danny is making originally are heavy: it puts a strain on

his relationship with Vicky, it makes him feel stressed out in general, it makes him angry with Vicky. The benefits are few: possibly it might make Vicky a bit more cautious about what she says in future, but does Danny really want her to be nervous about everything she says? A better appraisal would be something like the 'best friend' said in (2) above. That would have lots of benefits for Danny and no costs.

And another one . . .

Exercise

When thirteen-year-old Nathaniel accidentally dropped a mug on the kitchen floor and it broke, his mother Lola 'completely lost it'. Her appraisal was that 'The kid is spoiled to death, he just doesn't realise that things cost money, he just doesn't give a damn. He thinks I'll clear up after him, buy everything that's necessary and just act as his slave. Well, it's about time he learned a lesson.' Again. . .

1. What errors in thinking is Lola making?
2. What alternative appraisal would an all-knowing, all-wise friend suggest?

3. How might Lola reframe what Nathaniel did?
4. What would a cost–benefit analysis of Lola's appraisal look like? Can you suggest a better appraisal?

And again you are probably best to work the answers out yourself before going on to read the ones below.

1. Lola is using emotive language ('he doesn't give a damn, he thinks I'll act like his slave, it's about time he learned a lesson'), she is mind-reading (how does she know he doesn't give a damn?) and she is probably overgeneralising (just because he drops the occasional mug it doesn't mean he doesn't care about things or that he sees his mother as a slave).
2. An all-knowing, all-wise friend might say, 'Listen, Lola, how much does a mug cost? And is it really that difficult to sweep up a broken mug? In any case, you could get him to do that, and that would probably be the best way of him "learning a lesson", as you put it. Now, just calm yourself down and get him to clear up the bits.'
3. Possibly Lola might reframe the incident as another small part of Nathaniel's development, in that he learns that when you make a mistake, even a small one, like breaking a mug, you have to rectify it – in this case, sweep up the pieces.

Or she could look at it from a completely different perspective: she could take the view of one of the millions of people in the world whose lives are seriously at risk on a daily basis and then ask herself how one such person would perceive the breaking of a mug that was easily replaced.

4. A cost–benefit analysis of Lola's appraisal would be that the costs to her are heavy: she is stressed-out, agitated, angry with Nathaniel and wearing down the relationship between them. The benefits of such an appraisal are slim: possibly Nathaniel might be somewhat more careful next time, but it's equally possible he may be so nervous next time he is in the kitchen with his mum that he is more likely to drop something; or perhaps he might not even risk making himself a drink when she's about, so she would see less of him around the house. Again, a better appraisal would be that of the best friend or even possibly that [in (3) above] of a person whose life is constantly at risk on a daily basis, i.e. 'a broken mug is nothing to worry about'.

So how do you change really, permanently?

The RCR technique

RCR stands for *Review, Consolidate, Record*. And each of these is very important.

Reviewing means you examine events that happen to you (and especially events when you have felt angry and irritable) in exactly the same way as we have done in the three exercises we have just looked at. In other words, you actually write down what happened to you in exactly the same way as in each of these exercises. The description can be quite brief; it need only take up a few lines. Importantly, though, it does contain both the event and your appraisal of it – just like the examples. And again, just as in the exercises, you take yourself through the four stages of analysis. Use Diary 2 if it helps.

The purpose of this is for you to form a judgement as to how you should best view the event. Now, you might say that you can't *decide* how to view an event – an event happens and your appraisal/judgement appears in a flash and is therefore the true one. A lot of us feel this; but I'm afraid it is the thinking of a five-year-old: 'Because I see it this way it *is* this way.' Not at all. Events happen, and there are as many different ways of seeing them as there are people in the world. What you have to do is come to a judgement as to your best way of seeing it, the way that is in your best interests.

This can be tricky, because by now you will certainly be well into the habit of seeing things in particular ways, and changing those ways is quite a task. Rather like finding your way through a jungle, it is always easier to take the already existing paths. However, it is unfortunate for you if those paths happen to be 'the all or nothing path', 'the emotive language path', 'the mind-reading path' and so on.

There is some good news, though: as far as the brain is concerned it doesn't really matter much whether you do things in reality or in imagination. What this means is that simply reviewing things in the way I have just described, taking yourself through the four stages of analysis, and simply *imagining* thinking in the most cost-effective way is almost as good as actually doing it at the time of the event in terms of changing your patterns of thinking. Nevertheless, you do have to do it lots of times. Effectively, you are beating a new path through the jungle of the brain; and you have to keep treading down that path to make it a viable route. So keep reviewing, keep taking yourself through the four stages, and keep settling on the most cost-effective appraisal.

(For those of you who watch cricket, you will sometimes see a batsman rehearsing the stroke *he should have played*. On the face of it this seems a pretty daft thing to do, as the ball has just gone whistling past him and he played a poorer stroke than the one he is now rehearsing. Not so, however: that rehearsal he is now doing is in fact treading down a better path through the jungle of the brain. The next time a cricket ball comes towards him in similar fashion there is a better chance that he will take that new improved path rather than the previous faulty one. For those of you who are not interested in cricket, you must wonder what on earth I am talking about. Don't worry. Think jungle.)

Consolidating is equally important. Just as it's impossible to distinguish between the relative importance of brakes and steering on a car, so it is with reviewing and consolidating. They are both essential.

What you do with consolidating is act out the appraisal you settled on during the review stage. In other words, thinking something is not enough; you actually have to *behave* that way. I call it consolidating simply because it consolidates the thoughts you have produced. Thoughts and behaviour make a very strong combination – indeed, this is the key combination that underlies a cognitive behavioural approach to solving problems.

So, in the examples given in the exercises above, Lemy must 'act out' being pleased that Ella feels secure enough in the relationship that she can have a great time laughing and joking with other men. This is more than simply pretending, because by now Lemy really has reframed the situation and has got his new cost-effective appraisal; so it is a question of 'acting out what he thinks' rather than pretending. In other words, he would joke with Ella about it all afterwards, might tease her about it while it is going on, and so on.

Likewise, Danny will genuinely act out his new more cost-effective appraisal to the slip-ups that Vicky makes. So he can tease her about how her mouth runs away with her, the new perception that other people have of him, and so forth.

Lola, too, will consolidate her new appraisal by *calmly* asking Nathaniel to sweep up the remnants of the mug, in due course *calmly* buy a replacement mug or two, and so on.

Importantly, this need not just be retrospective. Lemy can be sure that he reacts this way to *future* flirting episodes from Ella; Danny can be sure he reacts this way to *future* misjudged comments from Vicky; and Lola should ensure that she reacts this way to *future* 'careless acts' from Nathaniel.

Recording is the part where you reap the pay-off: now you can simply enjoy feeling pleased with yourself. All you do is write down a brief account of events as they happen; so, Danny will simply make a brief note about Vicky's latest gaffe, what his new, improved appraisal was, and how he reacted during it and afterwards. And Lola will do just the same, keeping an account of the things that Nathaniel gets up to, her new appraisals and her new reactions.

So the recording stage is clearly the most fun and enables you to see that your hard work is paying off in a good way: not just that those around you are not having to suffer your irritability and anger, but that you are genuinely seeing things in a different light, one which is more beneficial for you too.

Summary

- The reason why you get irritated and angry at things that don't seem to bother other people is that you make different appraisals and judgements about those events.

- The most common errors made in appraising and judging situations are selective perception, mind-reading, all or nothing thinking, using emotive language and overgeneralisation.
- It is straightforward – with lots of practice – to analyse examples and see the errors that are being made.
- It is possible to make appraisals and judgements that are better for all concerned, making both you and other people feel better about the situation. The main ways of doing this are:

    (a) identify the thinking error and correct it, (b) the 'friend technique' (how will an all-knowing, all-wise friend advise you to view the situation?), (c) reframe the situation by searching for good aspects of it or viewing it from a completely different perspective, and (d) conduct a cost–benefit analysis, examining the costs and benefits of appraising the situation the way you are doing and then looking for a more cost-effective way.

- You can bring about a permanent change in your own behaviour by the RCR technique. This means reviewing events as they crop up and conducting the four-stage analysis to produce more helpful appraisals and judgements, consolidating this new, more cost-effective appraisal by behaving in a way that matches it, then recording the results to further consolidate the gains and generally make you feel good about your progress.

Project

The best project you can carry out to apply this chapter to your own situation, and thereby change your own behaviour, is as follows:

- Keep a record of events that trigger your anger and, most importantly, what your appraisal of those events is. Use Diary 2 if you want; there are more copies in the appendix.
- Analyse your appraisals and produce better, more helpful, more cost-effective ones. A brief account of how to do this is contained in the fourth point of the summary above.
- Consolidate your new appraisals by acting in line with them. This is a strong technique

where your thoughts and behaviour support each other.

It is a good idea also to record in writing what you have just done (the trigger, your new appraisal, how you acted on that new appraisal); this consolidates things even further.

13

Do yourself a favour: give yourself some good advice

Time for a different type of intervention. In this one there is no writing involved!

It is based on a study reported by Prof. Sofia Osimo at the University of Barcelona. Hers was a rather complicated study in which the subjects wore 3-D glasses and saw avatars of themselves and of themselves looking like Sigmund Freud. Then she contrived to have the subjects, appearing to be Sigmund Freud, giving themselves advice. Well we are not going to manage anything quite as ambitious as that, but we can do what I think is equally good, very simply.

There is a long history of 'chair work', some of which gets quite complicated too, but it doesn't need to be like that, so this is what I suggest.

The first thing we know is that it generally works well if we give ourselves advice. So, you can if you like give yourself some advice about your irritability and anger. For example, you might – in your current tranquil state – advise yourself on the best way of becoming less irritable and less angry in future. And the chances are this would work well for you. (I wouldn't do it when you are in a rage because there is a risk that the emotional part of the brain hijacks the rest of the brain and urges you to do things you'd be ill-advised to do. This is not advice; it is your emotional brain urging you to let it have its way!) So always wait until you have cooled down and the chances are that this will be effective. But there are several things you can do to strengthen this effect – to make it even more powerful.

The first is to find yourself two chairs and to sit in one of them and describe your problem out loud to the other chair, imagining that somebody is sitting there. Then you move over to the second chair and give yourself some advice, again out loud, talking to the first chair as though you are still there. Depending on how self-conscious you are, you might like to do it when there is nobody else around!

Why do we bother with two chairs? The answer is that while you are sitting in the first chair you can concentrate on describing exactly what the problem is, then, when you are in the second chair you can concentrate on describing exactly what you think would be the best solution – the best advice to give. The separation of the two chairs helps us to separate problem from advice whereas when we are trying to think things through normally, just quietly in our minds, the two get hopelessly entangled with each other rather like two different colours of plasticine being rolled up together and producing some horrible amalgamation that is neither one thing nor the other.

The interesting thing that Prof. Osimo found was that people gave themselves better advice when they were 'pretending to be' Sigmund Freud. This is curious because none of the subjects had any specialist knowledge of Sigmund Freud, so I suspect what was happening was that they imagined that Freud would probably give them considered, compassionate advice and so proceeded to give themselves just that. More considered and more compassionate than when they were simply being themselves.

So, the obvious improvement you can make is that when you go in the second chair to give yourself some advice you simply pretend you are Sigmund Freud while you do it, because we know that people tend to give themselves better advice when they are 'pretending to be' Freud. I think this is a fascinating thing because the advice is obviously coming from yourself but is actually better advice than when you are simply being yourself! Even so, it will be good advice because you know everything you need to know about the problem and your feelings on it – even things you might not tell a therapist.

So you could stop there, and the chances are you would be doing very well for yourself. I love this technique because it is so simple and tends to work so well. Moreover, once you get over the self-consciousness of it, it can be fun.

But you can enhance it still further if you want, and whether you will want to or not probably depends on how much you like gadgets. This is because the simplest way of enhancing it is to record each stage, for example on your smartphone, then play it back to yourself.

So the final deluxe version is like this:

1. You sit in the first chair and describe your problem to an imaginary person sitting in the second chair, recording what you say.
2. You move to the second chair, place the recorder on the first chair and play back the recording. Whilst listening to the recording you imagine yourself to be Sigmund Freud or maybe some other wise and compassionate person.
3. Having listened to the problem, and still in your role as Sigmund Freud and still sitting in the second chair, you give advice to the first chair, again recording this advice.
4. You move back to the first chair, so being yourself again, and play back the recording of the advice. Because you are sitting in the first chair, you are receptive to this advice, inclined to take it on board and to act on it.

So, whether you go for the simplest version, the most deluxe version, or the one in the middle, the following rules apply:

*   When you are in chair one you are either describing the problem or being receptive to advice.
*   When you are in chair two you are either listening to the problem or giving advice.

Finally, there are several tips which make it as good as can be:

1. You only get one shot at describing the problem and hearing the advice. This means that when you are sitting in chair one listening to the advice you can't reply to chair two – and in particular you can't say 'yes but that wouldn't work because . . .' You can only listen to the advice.

2. You can use this technique as many times as you like over the weeks, months and years. It's a great technique and is useful in all sorts of situations. However, don't use it more than once per day otherwise you get into the scenario above where you start arguing with the advice that you gave yourself earlier on.

3. The advice that you give yourself can be anything. For example, it needn't correspond to anything that you have read in this book so far (although it can do if you like). It may be very down-to-earth (for example: 'If I were you I'd make sure you eat better, drink less, get more exercise and get a good night's sleep every night' or it may be more sophisticated, for example addressing thinking errors. Have faith in yourself because the chances are you will give yourself advice that is very useful for you.

Project

The project here is self-evident – try it out! Better still, try it out a few times because, even though it seems very simple, you quickly get better at it and it quickly becomes more fun.

Incidentally, in the jargon of the profession, this kind of technique is known as 'a higher order technique' simply because the kind of advice you end up giving yourself is of a higher order than any prescribed advice that you might receive from elsewhere. The two-chair technique allows you to access advice that is otherwise difficult to access.

Taking it further

If you want to see me demonstrating chair work, go to YouTube and search for 'chair work William Davies' and it shall be yours.

14

Why do I get angry?
2: beliefs

We have covered a great deal of ground so far, and if you have acted on it you will already have made a terrific impact on your own irritability and anger. Nevertheless, there is a question that might have occurred to you, and it is a question that can appear in several forms, as follows:

- Why is it always me who makes these unhelpful appraisals and judgements, rather than my friend Joe, Kate or whoever?
- Why was it Omar who got angry about the guy who came into the bar and left the door open, rather than Carlos or Ryan?
- Why was it that Lola made the unhelpful appraisal/judgement when her son dropped her mug on the floor, whereas other mothers don't make such unhelpful appraisals?
- Why did Amy make such an unhelpful appraisal of her twelve-year-old who was washing her

---

> hair in the bath (not tidying her room) while some other mothers wouldn't?
>
> • Why is it that when Chris is 'cut up' by another motorist, he makes an appraisal that gets him really angry, whereas other motorists will just shrug it off?

Of course, these are all simply different forms of the same question: namely, why are some people 'set up' to make unhelpful appraisals whereas other people seem to be set up to make helpful appraisals?

We talked about this in Part One, so in this chapter we will look at how to remedy the situation. If you are someone who is prone to making unhelpful appraisals, appraisals which lead you to be irritable and angry quite often, then this is your chance to re-programme yourself. And, perhaps surprisingly, it's not too difficult.

Let's go back to our model. We can see from the diagram that the way we appraise things is influenced partly by our beliefs. We've shaded that box in because that's the box we're going to focus on in this chapter. We are going to look at how those beliefs influence the way we appraise things and how we can alter those beliefs; because if we can do that, then we will automatically alter our appraisals without any further effort. We will, effectively, be a significantly different person, someone who is fundamentally less prone to be irritable and angry.

You can see from the Figure 14.1 that by changing the beliefs we will change the whole course of events.

Incidentally, you might be thinking that it's not so much that you are *always* prone to making unhelpful appraisals; it's just that *sometimes* you are. Particularly when you just 'feel irritable'. In that case, Chapter 23 on 'mood' is going to be especially relevant to you. Even so, if you are wondering whether it's worth your while reading this chapter (and all the others between here and the mood chapter) then I would suggest that the most likely answer is: 'Yes, it is.' This one in particular is just such a good chapter! It looks at things which are absolutely fundamental and yet relatively easy to change. So, potentially there is a big pay-off for little effort, and pleasurable effort at that.

What sort of beliefs are we talking about?

What we are dealing with here are beliefs about yourself, about other people, about the nature of the world, about how things should be, about how life is to be lived, and so on. We are *not* concerned with beliefs on matters of fact (as in, I believe it is about 3,500 miles from London to New York, or I believe the capital of Australia is Canberra).

A lot has been written about the beliefs that people hold and how helpful or otherwise they are (especially by Aaron T Beck and Albert Ellis). People have made lists of unhelpful beliefs – beliefs that make you anxious, beliefs that make you depressed, and so forth. In my experience, having read lots of lists and seen lots of irritable and angry people, my own list of unhelpful beliefs is as follows:

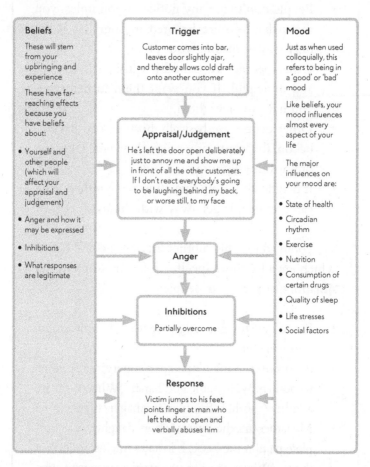

Beliefs

These will stem from your upbringing and experience

These have far-reaching effects because you have beliefs about:

- Yourself and other people (which will affect your appraisal and judgement)

- Anger and how it may be expressed

- Inhibitions

- What responses are legitimate

Trigger

Customer comes into bar, leaves door slightly ajar, and thereby allows cold draft onto another customer

Appraisal/Judgement

He's left the door open deliberately just to annoy me and show me up in front of all the other customers. If I don't react everybody's going to be laughing behind my back, or worse still, to my face

Anger

Inhibitions

Partially overcome

Response

Victim jumps to his feet, points finger at man who left the door open and verbally abuses him

Mood

Just as when used colloquially, this refers to being in a 'good' or 'bad' mood

Like beliefs, your mood influences almost every aspect of your life

The major influences on your mood are:

- State of health
- Circadian rhythm
- Exercise
- Nutrition
- Consumption of certain drugs
- Quality of sleep
- Life stresses
- Social factors

Figure 14.1 A model for analysing irritability and anger

- Things should be just exactly how I want them to be. It is awful if they are not.
- People don't take any notice of you unless you show that you are irritated or angry. It is the only way of making your point.
- Other people are basically selfish, self-centred and unhelpful. If you want them to help you, you have to *make* them.
- Other people are basically hostile. You have to be on the alert, otherwise they will take any opportunity to put you down.
- If people do wrong they must be punished. You can't let people get away with things.

We could add to this another list of unhelpful beliefs which are a bit more specific, referring to particular situations or particular people:

- It's okay to get angry with/hit policemen, bouncers, etc.
- A parent/foreman/manager/supervisor is *meant* to be snappy, irritable and harsh. (Where you are a father/mother/foreman/manager/supervisor.)
- My father/mother/partner/son/daughter is a complete pain in the neck, it irritates me just to look at them. (Where there is one particular person who produces that emotional reaction in you.)

Exercise

Let's have a look at the basic list of five unhelpful beliefs. In each of the following examples, underline the answer you think is best. In some cases there may be more than one possibility; in those cases underline more than one. The first two have been completed for you.

1. Omar, Carlos and Ryan are all sitting in a bar, near to the door. During the course of the evening four people come in and leave the door open. When the fifth person comes in it is Omar who gets angry.

   This is because Omar believes that things should be just how he wants them / <u>believes people take no notice unless you are irritated or angry</u> / <u>believes people are selfish, self-centred and unhelpful</u> / believes people are hostile and constantly trying to put you down / believes if people do wrong they must be punished, you can't let people get away with things.

2. In a particular street in a medium-sized town there are seventeen mothers who have youngsters between the ages of five and fifteen. All those youngsters, to a greater or lesser degree, drop mugs on the floor from time to time.

   Lola gets much angrier than any of the other sixteen because <u>she believes that things should be just how she wants them</u> / <u>believes people take no notice unless you are irritated or angry</u> / believes people are selfish, self-centred and unhelpful / believes people are hostile and constantly trying to put you down / believes if people do wrong they must be punished, you can't let people get away with things.

3. Errol's wife has a habit of contradicting him when they are out in public. This makes him very angry because he feels he 'loses face' in front of other people.

   This is because he basically believes that things should be just how he wants them / believes people take no notice unless you are irritated or angry / believes people are selfish, self-centred and unhelpful / believes people are hostile and constantly trying to put you down / believes if people do wrong they must be punished, you can't let people get away with things.

4. Brandon, the electrician, feels really 'put upon' and angry when his boss asks him to do extra tasks towards the end of the day.

   He tends to see his boss in this light because he basically believes that things should be just how he wants them / believes people take no notice unless you are irritated or angry / believes people are selfish, self-centred and unhelpful / believes people are hostile and constantly trying to put you down / believes if people do wrong they must be punished, you can't let people get away with things.

5. When Ella laughs and jokes with other men it makes her husband, Lemy, very angry. On the other hand,

when Michelle laughs and jokes with other men, her husband Jamie does not get angry. The difference between the two men is that Lemy basically believes that things should be just how he wants them / believes people take no notice unless you are irritated or angry / believes people are selfish, self-centred and unhelpful / believes people are hostile and constantly trying to put you down / believes if people do wrong they must be punished, you can't let people get away with things.

6. One evening in November 1999 a total of around one million people drank in a British bar. Of that one million people, about 10,000 were jogged so that they spilt their drink over themselves. Of those 10,000, Terry was the only one who broke a beer mug and pushed it in the face of the person who jogged him.

   Part of the reason he reacted so badly is that he believes that things should be just how he wants them / believes people take no notice unless you are irritated or angry / believes people are selfish, self-centred and unhelpful / believes people are hostile and constantly trying to put you down / believes if people do wrong they must be punished, you can't let people get away with things.

7. On a particular estate in a particular city there are around six hundred children between the ages of five and fifteen. Only about fifty of them keep their

rooms tidy enough to satisfy their parents. Most parents on this estate nag their children to keep their rooms tidier. Amy, on the other hand, completely 'loses her cool' with her twelve-year-old daughter.

This is because Amy believes that things should be just how she wants them / believes people take no notice unless you are irritated or angry / believes people are selfish, self-centred and unhelpful / believes people are hostile and constantly trying to put you down / believes if people do wrong they must be punished, you can't let people get away with things.

8. Aaron feels terrible because he hit his twelve year-old son across the face because the boy hadn't done his homework and had lied to him about it.

   However, Aaron was prone to react this way because deep down he believes that things should be just how he wants them / believes people take no notice unless you are irritated or angry / believes people are selfish, self-centred and unhelpful / believes people are hostile and constantly trying to put you down / believes if people do wrong they must be punished, you can't let people get away with things.

9. Another driver cut across Chris' path as he was going round a roundabout. He got so angry that he 'tailgated' the other driver for five miles. Eventually, the other driver got out and confronted Chris, and there was a fight during which Chris came off very much second best.

Chris would never have behaved this way in the first place had he not believed that things should be just how he wants them / believed people take no notice unless you are irritated or angry / believed people are selfish, self-centred and unhelpful / believed people are hostile and constantly trying to put you down / believed if people do wrong they must be punished, you can't let people get away with things.

How did you get on? Below is the same list of my own answers. Some of them are certainly debatable, but at least they will give you food for thought.

1. Omar, Carlos and Ryan are all sitting in a bar, near to the door. During the course of the evening four people come in and leave the door open. When the fifth person comes in it is Omar who gets angry.

   This is because Omar believes people are selfish, self-centred and unhelpful and that you can't let people get away with things.

2. In a particular street in a medium-sized town there are seventeen mothers who have youngsters between the ages of five and fifteen. All those youngsters, to a greater or lesser degree, drop mugs on the floor from time to time.

   Lola gets much angrier than any of the other sixteen because she believes that things should be just how she wants them and that people take no notice unless you are irritated or angry.

3. Errol's wife has a habit of contradicting him when they are out in public. This makes him very angry because he feels he 'loses face' in front of other people.

   This is because he believes people are hostile and constantly trying to put you down.

4. Brandon, the electrician, feels really 'put upon' and angry when his boss asks him to do extra tasks towards the end of the day.

   He tends to see his boss in this light because he believes people are selfish, self-centred and unhelpful.

5. When Ella laughs and jokes with other men it makes her husband, Lemy, very angry. On the other hand, when Michelle does the same thing, her husband Jamie does not get angry. The difference between the two men is that Lemy basically believes that things should be just how he wants them and that people are hostile and constantly trying to put you down.

6. One evening in November 1999 a total of around one million people drank in a British bar. Of that one million people about 10,000 were jogged so that they spilt their drink over them. Of those 10,000, Terry was the only one who broke a beer mug and pushed it in the face of the person who jogged him.

   Part of the reason he reacted so badly is that he believes that people are hostile and constantly trying to put you down, and that if people do wrong they must be punished, you can't let people get away with things.

7. On a particular estate in a particular city there are around six hundred children between the ages of five and fifteen. Only about fifty of them keep their rooms tidy enough to satisfy their parents. Most parents on this estate nag their children to keep their rooms tidier. Amy, on the other hand, completely 'loses her cool' with her twelve-year-old daughter.

   This is because Amy believes that things should be just how she wants them, that people take no notice unless you are irritated or angry and believes if people do wrong they must be punished, you can't let people get away with things.

8. Aaron feels terrible because he hit his twelve year-old son across the face because the boy hadn't done his homework and had lied to him about it.

   However, Aaron was prone to react this way because he believes people take no notice unless you are irritated or angry and that if people do wrong they must be punished, you can't let people get away with things.

9. Another driver cut across Chris' path as he was going round a roundabout. He got so angry that he 'tail-gated' the other driver for five miles. Eventually, the other driver got out and confronted Chris, and there

was a fight during which Chris came off very much second best.

Chris would never have behaved this way in the first place had he not believed that people are hostile and constantly trying to put you down and that if people do wrong they must be punished, you can't let people get away with things.

And you can see the terrific pay-off that each of these people would receive if only they could alter their beliefs. For example:

1. Not only would Omar not be angry when somebody leaves the bar door open, he would not get so angry when somebody gets served ahead of him in the queue, when Carlos doesn't buy a round of drinks when it's his turn, etc. (Importantly, this is not to say that Omar will not rectify these things, just that he won't get angry about it.)

2. Lola will not only remain calm when her son drops a mug on the floor, she would also remain calm when he forgets to take an essential item to school. (Again, this is not to say that she would not try and develop his taking more care over things.)

3. If Errol could change his beliefs he would feel much easier about his wife contradicting him in public because he wouldn't anticipate a critical reaction from other people. Equally, he would feel much

more relaxed in a whole host of social situations for exactly the same reason.

4. If Brandon, the electrician, could alter his belief that other people are always likely to be trying to take advantage of him, then he would feel less put upon when his boss asks him to do extra jobs. Equally, he would feel more relaxed in other situations too.

5. If Lemy could realise that other people (including his wife Ella, and the men she flirts with) are not always trying to put you down, he would feel much more relaxed about her playfulness. Equally, he would feel much more relaxed in a whole host of other situations.

6. The same applies to Terry. His belief that other people are hostile and likely to be putting you down resulted in very serious consequences for him when he put a broken beer mug in the face of the person who jogged his elbow. Not only could those consequences have been avoided but, had he realised that most people are not hostile in this way, he would have lived a much more relaxed and enjoyable life.

7. Amy got extremely angry with her twelve-year-old daughter because she didn't tidy her room, and Amy believes that things have got to be the way she wants, and that people take no notice unless you get angry with them. She too would be leading a much more enjoyable life if she could accept that, by and large,

things tend not to be quite how you would like them to be, but that this *doesn't really matter*. And anyway, people 'develop better' with constructive interactions rather than by getting angry with them.

8. A similar kind of thing applies to Aaron, who hit his twelve-year-old son across the face. If Aaron could get to realise that it's not the end of the world if things aren't just how he wants them to be and that's it's probably not true that people take no notice unless you get really angry with them, he wouldn't have done this. Equally, he stands to benefit in all sorts of situations if he can remedy those beliefs.

9. Things worked out very badly for Chris after somebody cut across his path on a roundabout and he eventually came to grief in a fight with the other driver. If only he hadn't believed that people must be punished if they do something wrong he could have avoided this. But again, this is only one example of Chris constantly giving himself a bad time because he believed that. Equally, he stands to benefit in all sorts of situations if he can remedy those beliefs.

Developing more helpful beliefs

For this we use the AA method – which, in this case, has nothing to do with too much alcohol consumption. Here it stands simply for (a) developing better Alternative beliefs and (b) Acting them out.

Here are some suggestions:

- Unhelpful belief: Things should be just exactly how I want them to be. It is awful if they are not.
- Suggestion for more helpful alternative: It's nice if things are just the way I want them, but it's not the end of the world if they're not.
- Unhelpful belief: People don't take any notice of you unless you show that you are irritated or angry. It is the only way of making your point.
- Suggestion for more helpful alternative: Although you can sometimes get people to do what you want by being irritable and angry with them, you never really get them on your side. So it's better to talk and persuade. Even then people won't always do what we want, but that's not the end of the world either.
- Unhelpful belief: Other people are basically selfish, self-centred and unhelpful. If you want them to help you, you have to *make* them.
- Suggestion for more helpful alternative: Although there are some people who are very selfish indeed, most people will help each other out if asked.
- Unhelpful belief: Other people are basically hostile. You have to be on the alert otherwise they will take any opportunity to put you down.

- Suggestion for more helpful alternative: Although there are a few people who can be quite hostile, most people basically support one another and take a good view of each other.
- Unhelpful belief: If people do wrong they must be punished, you can't let people get away with things.
- Suggestion for more helpful alternative: It's better to persuade than punish, to look to the future rather than the past. Sometimes you can't even persuade and people do get away with things. So, I'll just keep up my own standards.
- Unhelpful belief: It's okay to get angry with/hit policemen, bouncers, etc.
- Suggestion for more helpful alternative: Policemen, bouncers etc. are actually real people just like anybody else. It's no more reasonable to hit them than to hit any other person.
- Unhelpful belief: A father/mother/foreman/manager/supervisor is *meant* to be snappy, irritable and harsh. (Where you are a father/mother/foreman/manager/ supervisor.)
- Suggestion for more helpful alternative: A father/mother/foreman/manager/ supervisor needs to set a good example. That means being friendly and supportive rather than irritable and angry.
- Unhelpful belief: My father/mother/partner/son/daughter is a complete pain in the neck,

> it irritates me just to look at him/her. (Where there is one particular person who produces that emotional reaction in you.)
>
> • Suggestion for more helpful alternative: My father/ mother/partner/son/daughter is just like anybody else – they've got their good points and bad points. It's no use getting hung up on their bad points.

Use cue-cards if you want

Some people actually write out a small card for themselves (known as a cue-card). This has the unhelpful belief written on the one side and a more helpful alternative on the other. Sometimes people will make quite elaborate versions of these. For example, you might write the unhelpful version in red (for 'danger') and the more helpful version on the other side in green (for 'go'). And you might perhaps add an exhortation after the helpful version, like 'Now do it!' Some people even go off to their local print shop and get the card nicely laminated once they have got it just how they want! Whether you like your card basic or exotic, it's quite a nice idea to carry it around with you as a constant reminder. You probably won't need eight cards – it's unlikely that you are falling prey to all eight of the unhelpful beliefs, probably just one or two – in which case you just need one or two cards.

You could also do something similar on your phone or as a pop-up on a computer.

Acting it out

You will probably remember that we noted in the previous chapter that *thinking* differently is not enough. You also need to *act* on your new thoughts. New thoughts and new behaviour make a terrifically powerful combination. Rather in the way that two bicycles can lean against each other and prop each other up in a perfectly stable way for ever, your new thinking is supported by your new behaviour and, equally, your new behaviour is supported by your new thinking. The two will constantly reinforce each other. It's the closest we are ever going to get to perpetual motion.

So how do we act it out? There are a couple of possibilities:

- Simply imagine how a person with the new, more helpful alternative belief would act and mimic that.
- Find yourself a role model. In other words, think of somebody who acts like they believe the new improved belief, imagine what they would do, and do it.

In either case you have to do it with a degree of conviction. For example, Lola of the mug-dropping teenage son needs to really work on her belief that he is basically okay (rather than fundamentally selfish), and she would do well to set an example of friendliness and helpfulness and really act like she *believes* these two new beliefs. So, rather than uttering the words 'Get a brush and sweep it up' through clenched teeth (which, admittedly would be an improvement over her previous behaviour), she goes the whole hog and says, 'Get a brush and sweep it up, there's a good boy', complete with matching encouraging tone. The point is that what she is aiming for is not simply to tidy up her behaviour so that it's not so wearing for her and everybody else, but to align her new, more helpful behaviour with new, more helpful underlying beliefs, so that she is genuinely at peace with herself and other people can see that. This is clearly much better for all concerned than simply 'keeping the lid on it'.

In just the same way Omar, sitting near the door of the bar, will now realise that the five individuals who left the door open are not selfish scoundrels who deserve punishment, but perfectly okay individuals who just need to be reminded to shut the door. The way he asks them to do that will therefore be friendly and calm, in line with that belief. Likewise, Errol, whose wife contradicts him in public, will realise that although others might laugh when this happens, this does not indicate that they are fundamentally hostile to him, because people are mostly supportive and friendly. Acting it out, he can now join in the laughter. Similarly

Brandon need not get himself into a stew by distressing himself over things not being just as he would like them to be. He can simply get on and do the job the boss asks, or not. What was winding him up was how awful it was that things were not as he would wish. Now he's resigned to that fact he can simply get on with things. Ella's flirting need not irritate Lemy now that he accepts that neither Ella nor other people are basically hostile, but rather that most people are friendly and supportive; he can take Ella's behaviour for the harmless amusement it is, and act things out by just joining in.

Terry, too, had he accepted that most people are okay rather than hostile, would not have jumped to the conclusion that his elbow was jogged deliberately at the bar. He would have assumed it was an accident, possibly made a joke out of it, and might even have got himself a free pint. Amy would not have lost her temper with her daughter, sitting in the bath not tidying her room. Rather than being so uptight because things were not as she would wish (the room was still untidy) and determined that the girl must be punished for her misdemeanour, she could have accepted that sometimes children have untidy rooms and that anyway her best option is to be setting a good example as a parent. Nor need Chris have gone chasing the man who cut across his path on the roundabout. If only he had accepted that people do not need to be punished for their misdemeanours, and that sometimes they even get away with them, he could have simply acted this belief out by keeping up his own standards and driving his car as he thinks cars should be driven – and saved himself a lot of trouble.

A role model can be helpful

We can see from these examples that it is straightforward enough to decide on a new belief and act it out in daily life. Plenty of people do that with a lot of success and a lot of pleasure. (It is very satisfying to see yourself take charge of your own destiny, decide on sensible beliefs and act in line with them.) Other people get to exactly the same destination by a different route. They think of a particular person who seems to have the kind of beliefs we have spoken about and ask themselves, 'What would s/he do in this situation?' For some people, imagining it makes it a lot easier to mimic. And mimicking the behaviour effectively consolidates the new beliefs.

The role model can be somebody you know, like a friend or relative, or it can be somebody you've never actually met – someone you've seen on television, perhaps. One important point if you choose the latter: it doesn't particularly matter if the person resembles their screen persona in real life or not. For example, my two favourite role models are the television business troubleshooter Marius Harvey-Jones and ace cricket commentator Brian Johnston. Now, I've never met either of these good people, and for all I know they might have been quite different in private life from the genial characters they presented on television and radio. As a matter of fact, both gentlemen are, or were – Brian

Johnston sadly died a few years back – by all accounts much the same in private life as they appeared in public. But my point here is that it doesn't matter; for the purpose of a role model, it is the persona you recognise that is important.

Nor do your role models have to match you in age or gender, or anything else. All that is important is that you can ask yourself: 'What perspective would s/he have taken on this?' and 'How would s/he have behaved in this situation?' and so on. The fact that I never quite live up to either of my models doesn't matter either; they certainly have a good effect. The key thing is that if you find yourself a good role model s/he can lead you into behaving just how you would wish to.

Reviewing and recording

Just as in a previous chapter, reviewing and recording are great habits to get into in order to entrench your new and more helpful beliefs.

'Reviewing' is literally looking again at the situation that has just passed and replaying it. You may be in the happy situation where you can enjoy reviewing how well you behaved, how well you brought into play your new beliefs and meshed them with splendid new behaviour. In which case, terrific: enjoy every moment of it. And it's not just enjoyment, either; it is, as we said before, a very useful activity to review things that have gone right. When things go well you have a good template for future success, so it is useful to consolidate and examine that template. If you've handled a difficult situation well, with no irritability and anger, then go back over it, review it, enjoy the moment.

Equally, if you've handled a situation badly in your view, if you've given in to some unhelpful beliefs and matched them with irritable and angry behaviour, then simply replay the situation how you think it should have gone. Remember to think the more helpful beliefs, and envisage the more helpful behaviour. *That replaying of the situation the way you would have preferred it to have gone is an extremely good thing to do*; it makes it more likely that it will go that way next time. (But beware: it is rather unhelpful simply to replay your *wrong* handling of the situation. It's best to regard that as 'water under the bridge'.)

Summary

- In this chapter we have covered how our beliefs affect the way we appraise and judge a situation, and as a consequence how we behave in that situation.
- We have listed the most common unhelpful beliefs that affect people's perceptions of the situations in which they find themselves.
- We have listed the more helpful alternative beliefs to replace the unhelpful ones.

- We have looked at the method for replacing unhelpful beliefs with helpful ones. This involves the AA method: highlighting the Alternative helpful belief and Acting out the situation in line with those beliefs.
- We have looked at the importance of reviewing successes and consolidating them as templates for good future behaviour, and also of review- ing failures – but reminding ourselves how we would have preferred to act in the situation, so we are more likely to get it right next time

Project

- Get yourself a piece of paper and write down any of the unhelpful beliefs that you think apply to you.
- For each of them, write down the more help- ful belief. This might be a question of simply copying down what I've written above, or you might want to put it into your own words.
- Replay a recent situation where your unhelpful beliefs have led you to appraise a situation badly and react in an irritable and angry way. Replay how you would have seen the situation if you

had had your more helpful beliefs in place, and what you would have done. (For example, if you are Omar you would replay sitting at the bar by the door, now believing that people, even those who leave doors open, are basically okay, appraising the situation differently and asking, in a proper friendly way, each person to close the door). Make it a good vivid replay in your mind.

- Most important of all, practise your new beliefs, seeing every situation through the eyes of someone who has these new beliefs, or through the eyes of a role model you've settled on. Then match your behaviour to your new perceptions – just as Omar would do in the previous point.

- Each time you achieve your goal, review that success and enjoy the moment. Review how your new beliefs helped, and how your new behaviour was in line with those beliefs. If you 'let yourself down', review the incident the way you would have preferred it to have gone. Pretty soon you will have lots of 'good' reviews and not many of the other sort!

15

Cats, camels and recreation: anger

Daft title for a chapter. Never mind, you might as well read it because it could just be very relevant to yourself. For some people it will be spot-on.

Remember the model we're working on is trigger, appraisal/judgement, anger, inhibitions, response. What we are talking about in this chapter is the 'anger' box; and there are just three points to make about it.

Displacing anger

The first point is that *anger can be displaced*. This process is commonly known as 'kicking the cat' or 'always hurting the one you love'. For example, you may have a bad day at work, but think that it is a bad idea to get angry with your boss. What you do, therefore, is to come home and (metaphorically, of course!) kick the cat: in other words, take it out on whoever or whatever happens to be around. The strange thing is that whoever or whatever turns out to be on the receiving end of your anger does in fact seem to be very irritating at the time in question. You are not always aware that you are 'displacing' your anger from your boss at work on to your loved ones/cat at home.

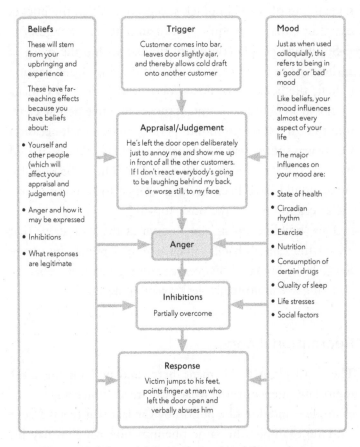

Figure 15.1 A model for analysing irritability and anger

Anger is additive

The second point is that *anger is additive*: it builds up. Again, the best analogy is the leaky bucket that we first used in Part One. Suppose you have a bucket with holes in it; it is still possible to fill the bucket to overflowing by pouring in several jugs of water in quick succession. When the bucket overflows, that's the equivalent of an outburst of anger.

So, if five people come into the bar within the space of an hour or two and each one leaves the door open causing a draft, the bucket overflows (or at least it does in Omar's case) and an outburst occurs. If those same five people came into the bar over a six-month period, and on each occasion Omar was sitting near the door, it is unlikely that he would have an outburst on the fifth occasion. This is because his anger would have been given a chance to 'leak away' on each occasion before the next 'top-up'.

This 'building up' is also known as the 'last straw that breaks the camel's back' phenomenon. I prefer the image of the leaky bucket, however, because, given half a chance, your anger will normally 'leak away' quite nicely.

Recreational anger

The third point to be made here, and perhaps the most important one, concerns what I call 'recreational anger'. An example – and don't be put off by the fact that this is a very extreme example; the same phenomenon happens day in, day out.

Very early on in my career, when I was working as a prison psychologist, I came across a prisoner who was having quite a lot of trouble serving his sentence; he got tense and agitated, and periodically smashed up his cell. I taught him how to relax and did some general 'counselling' work with him, with the result that he confided in me that he had been beaten up by half a dozen prison officers in the previous prison he had been held in. (I have no idea how true this allegation was, but that was what he told me.)

Anyway, he'd formed a plan that, on release, he would go and track down these six prison officers, and one by one shoot them.

I took this very seriously, (a) because I was young and naïve and took everything seriously, and (b) because he was already in prison for having shot somebody, so clearly he had the capability of doing what he said he was going to do. Furthermore he described how, on his previous sentence, he had done exactly the same thing: that is, he had spent time thinking and planning about how, when he got out, he would shoot this person. And, sure enough, he had done exactly that, and here he was back in prison again for that crime.

Now, it would be nice to think that young prison psychologists know exactly what to do in such a situation, but I didn't. So we simply got to talking around it, him telling me all about how it was . . .

To cut a long story short, he was in the habit of whiling away hour after hour fantasising about how he was going to get his revenge. This, apparently, was entirely pleasurable, and time flew by while he did this.

And this was the first case I came across of 'recreational anger': anger which at the very least passes the time of day, sometimes actually gives you a 'buzz' and often puts you into a different state of mind, so that actions which wouldn't normally seem sensible and rational look like they are. Going back to our leaky bucket analogy, it is as though you've plugged up all the holes in the bucket, keen to hang on to all the water there, and then just spent the time looking at the water. Or, rather more literally, you do everything to prevent your anger from drifting away and spend time dwelling and brooding about it.

The best course of action to take in this situation is as follows:

- Don't do whatever your anger is telling you to do.
- Do something else (more of which shortly).

Let's expand on that a little. When you are very irritable and angry it is as though that anger takes you over. The anger actually tells you to do things that, in your normal state, you wouldn't do. So who are you going to take more notice of, your anger or you yourself?

Well, the answer is obvious: it's more important to be true to yourself than to some temporary state of anger. On the other hand, it is very difficult simply to *refrain* from doing something. Rather like 'not thinking of a giraffe', it is virtually impossible. If someone tells you *not* to think of a giraffe, a picture of a long dappled neck springs to mind no matter how carefully you try to obey. In the same way, not to do what your anger tells you is very tricky indeed.

Getting away from anger

The answer is to *concentrate on doing something else*. Anything. Real-life examples of alternatives that people turn to in this situation include the following:

- Take physical exercise: walk, run, swim, etc.
- Read a book, magazine, newspaper.
- Watch television or listen to the radio.
- Go and do some gardening.
- Phone up or go and see a friend.
- Simply take yourself out of the situation and go somewhere else.

All of these are equivalent to 'doing something else'. And that is sufficient for most of us. In the case of the prisoner I was just telling you about, tactics such as reading a book would not be sufficient, because he had a long-term problem, ten times the size of anything afflicting most of us. Nevertheless, with him, we adopted exactly the same strategy, and he did indeed 'do something else'. He got in touch with a woman who ran a hostel for ex-prisoners and wrote to her to see whether that was somewhere he could stay after release.

Thank goodness, she wrote back telling him that might well be an option and, most importantly, included a photograph of the actual hostel (this was before the days of the internet!). I am sure it was that photograph that really persuaded him. Now he could literally envisage what else he could do upon leaving prison. Rather than going up to his previous prison and slowly stalking the six prison officers concerned, he could catch a train to this hostel and settle there. Happily, it was in a totally different part of the country.

Well, all that sounds very sensible, doesn't it? So why don't people do it? When you feel really angry and your anger is telling you to do something drastic, why do you sometimes do it even though the rational part of you knows that this is a temporary state you're in?

I think one of the reasons is that some people think it is more 'honest' to give vent to their anger. I don't agree. 'Honesty' is a splendid characteristic when it means (a) not lying or (b) not stealing from other people, but a very destructive characteristic when it is used to mean (c) saying tactless and hurtful things on the grounds that 'I'm only being honest' or (d) giving vent to angry urges without any thought of the consequences for yourself or other people. However we might describe these things, they have nothing to do with honesty.

Give yourself time

There's one important reason why it is always sensible, first, to refrain from doing what your anger is telling you, and second, to do something else. This is because, once you have truly regained your emotional equilibrium, you can decide at leisure what you think is best to do about the situation, rather than letting your anger tell you.

An example. Lemy described to me how on one occasion he was so agitated by his wife Ella's laughing and joking with other men that, even while still at the party they were both attending, he was going through in his mind how he was going to leave Ella and, more particularly, how he was going to tell Ella about his decision. He was relishing, in a strange sort of way, how this would 'teach her a lesson' and how sorry she would be.

And it was more by luck than judgement that this did not come to pass. In the car going home he was 'sulking' but in fact still rehearsing what he was going to say and still enjoying the anticipated effect. At home, the sulk continued but, as I say, more by luck than judgement he decided to postpone the confrontation until the next morning and simply go to sleep for the time being. Happily, by the next morning sleep had worked its magic, anger had retreated to a back seat and, although the discussion was heated, it was not as vitriolic as it would have been the previous evening. So, by accident, Lemy had followed the formula: Don't do what your anger tells you, do something else (in this case, go to sleep).

Lemy is one of my favourite cases, for two reasons. First, there are lots of people like him, men who have allowed their anger to tell them what to do and whose marriages have disintegrated as a result. Second, in Lemy's case, he was able eventually to do a complete review of his judgements and beliefs, rather along the lines of that set out in the previous chapters, and ended up seeing things in a completely different light. The net result was that Ella's behaviour did not simply become 'not irritating'; it became an asset to their relationship once he realised that it was harmless, and, perhaps more to the point, that everybody else knew that it had no serious intent.

Summary

- In talking about anger there are three points to be made. First, it can be displaced so that, although it might be your boss who has caused your anger, your partner or somebody else actually receives it. Second, anger is additive by nature. Envisage your anger as water in a leaky bucket. If another jugful of anger arrives before the first jugful has been allowed to leak away, then your bucket is filling up. Eventually, if a third, fourth or fifth jugful arrives, the bucket might overflow, leading to an angry outburst. Third, there is such a thing as 'recreational anger', where you get a peculiar kind of buzz from simply dwelling upon your anger and what you're going to do about it.
- Probably the best analogy for anger is the 'leaky bucket'. If it is topped up too quickly, then yes, it can overflow; but given half a chance, anger will leak away over a period of time.

- No matter whether your anger is about to over-flow, or whether you're in a state of recreational anger, or anything else, the best policy is (a) don't allow your anger to tell you what to do and (b) do anything else. Only when you've gained a good sense of equilibrium should you decide what to do about the situation that prompted the anger.

- The use of a role model (a person you use as a good example), can be very powerful here. You can simply ask yourself 'What would X [your model] do right now?' Interestingly, your anger will fight back and tell you to get on with allowing it to have its head. Just put it on hold for a moment, and really get to imagining what your good role model would do in the given situation.

Project

- One of the most important lessons in this chapter has been how to differentiate between what your anger tells you to do and what you yourself want to do. So a relevant project is to work on becoming more aware of both of these 'voices'. What I mean is, next time you are feeling angry, work out (a) what your anger is telling you to do and (b) what your 'real self' would tell you to do.

- It's good to practise this in situations which make you only slightly angry. The reason for this is that when you are very angry the 'angry voice' shouts so loud that it drowns out your 'true self' voice. You therefore have to practise being attuned to your 'true self' voice in mild-anger situations so that, eventually, you can hear it even in high-anger situations. And remember, most of us want to be loyal to our true self rather than to what anger tells us to do.

16

Dwelling, brooding and ruminating: why winding yourself up is dangerous

I want to tell you two stories about people winding themselves up, and see if they ring any bells with you. Stories a bit like the prisoner who was planning to kill half a dozen prison officers, but a bit more commonplace than that.

The first is from a group of bus drivers I was talking to. They said that from time to time they will have an altercation with somebody who gets on the bus. Maybe the person hasn't quite got enough money to pay the full fare but still thinks they should be allowed to ride the bus, and doesn't like it when the bus driver insists that they should pay full fare just like everybody else. That kind of thing. So there is an altercation, the passenger eventually forks out the money then goes and sits at the back of the bus. All is well.

Except it isn't, because what happens then is that the passenger sits there 'winding himself up', maybe thinking that the bus driver had spoken to him disrespectfully, maybe thinking the bus driver had been overzealous in getting the full fare from him and he was determined to pay a little less, whatever. What happens then is that, as the person goes to leave the bus, he embarks on a fully blown confrontation with the driver, often a shouting match ensues, sometimes the driver has to defend himself physically.

This is strange, isn't it, because nothing has happened between the first altercation and the second one, except that the passenger is sitting at the back of the bus. But can you imagine what was going on in the passenger's mind? He was getting himself into a spiral. I was going to say a downward spiral but I don't think it is, I think it's an upward spiral. A spiral where he feels very energetic, very incensed, and very right. It's anger all right, and very intense anger, but in a strange sort of way it is also enjoyable. Because you feel so energised and so right. When else do you feel like that? Maybe never.

The second story is about a similar thing has happened to me first-hand. Years ago one of our customers for whom we provide training did a bad thing in terms of breaching copyright. It was certainly a bad thing, but my reaction was completely over the top. And, moreover, it went on for months. I wrote a vitriolic letter to which the customer replied, and I replied to that, and they replied to that, and I replied to that, and so on. It was almost like a hobby, but it was a great hobby because, like the guys I've told you about, I too felt very energised by it, very right, and was showing how I was a person not to be messed with.

Now, of course, I feel completely stupid ever to have got myself into such a state; 'I must've been crazy.' I tell myself. And in a way, this is more than just a metaphor, the thinking we get ourselves into in these states is very close to delusional. And when we come down from it we can see this very clearly, but, sadly, we can't see it while we are in the state!

If you yourself have never been in such a state, nor have ever seen anybody else in such a state, then you probably have trouble imagining what I'm talking about. If on the other hand you have been in such a state, or know somebody who has, then you're probably very relieved to see this condition described. It's anger all right, and quite an extreme form of anger which is rarely discussed or talked about. It's a very serious one though, because it can take you over for days or months. And, as we have seen, can have very severe ramifications for your life and for the lives of those around you.

So, what can we do about it? There are two things: preventative measures and remedial measures.

One important preventative measure is keeping your biology right. Getting enough sleep, getting some exercise, eating a good diet, being wary of mood-altering substances such as alcohol etc. All of these give us a fighting chance of regulating our emotions in a reasonable way.

Then there are remedial measures. In other words, assuming you can spot yourself in such a state, what can you do about it? The best answer is this: take your grievance to a 'court of arbitration'. I put those words in quotes because it is not literally a court of arbitration, but a person you voluntarily give these powers to. Perhaps I am putting it too grandly. Or perhaps not, because the point about the court of arbitration is you abide by what it says. So, you can choose who you talk to and ask advice from but you must abide by two rules:

1. You must describe the situation to that person fairly and fully. You mustn't try to influence their judgement.
2. You must accept the judgement – their advice. This is important because your own judgement is in a funny place, it is not what it usually is, so you are doing yourself a disservice if you rely upon it. That's why you are asking a trusted friend, and so you must defer to their judgement and not simply ask somebody else until you get an opinion that fits with your temporarily distorted view!

So who do you ask? It's probably best if you decide that right now, assuming you're currently in a normal frame of mind. What you are looking for is somebody whose judgement you trust, and somebody who is 'on your side' in the sense that they tend to see the world in the same sort of ways you do – they would normally agree with your way of looking at things. This is important because you want somebody who will give you advice that fits in with your values. The whole point of the procedure is to overrule your temporarily distorted perspective with your normal judgement; in your state of high anger you're not able to do that for yourself, and that's why you turn to a trusted other person.

What if you haven't got a trusted other person (and plenty of people haven't). You still have to get someone other than yourself to straighten out your temporary distorted viewpoint, and I suggest the best way of doing this is from a counsellor or therapist. And the best way of finding such a person is to go via your general practitioner. But, again, be open about everything, just as you would with a trusted friend.

17

Mindfulness

A lot has been written about Mindfulness over the last ten years or so and some of it is very helpful for us. In this chapter I want to show you which bits are indeed helpful, and how to use them to your benefit.

Of all the skills involved in Mindfulness there are three key ones as far as we are concerned. They are:

1. The ability to observe.
2. The ability to describe.
3. To do both of these non-judgementally or dispassionately.

The exercise that people often describe in order to learn these skills is eating a raisin. This isn't a particularly useful exercise for us (I'll tell you what is in a second), but if you want to do the exercise that everybody else does, you need to find yourself a raisin and eat it. You don't just eat it, however; you put it in your mouth and you notice everything about it. Even before putting it in your mouth you observe what it looks like and describe what it looks like, you observe what it feels like and describe what it feels like.

All the while doing so non-judgementally; in other words, you don't say, 'I don't much like the look of it', you simply say, 'It is small, about the size of a penny piece and it is a round ball-shaped object, but soft and wrinkled. It's kind of browny/black colour, a little bit hard, but kind of squishy.' Or whatever you want to say along those lines. Then you put it in your mouth and again observe and describe it. So you might say, 'It doesn't really taste of anything very much, but I can feel the wrinkles on it, and again it is still squishy, I can squash it against the roof of my mouth with my tongue' etc. Again, notice that this is being done non-judgementally. For example, you don't say, 'I quite like the taste of it' or 'I don't like the taste of it'.

I said this isn't a particularly useful exercise for us, and maybe I was hasty in saying that. Maybe it's a good training exercise, because it is important for us to get good at observing things and describing things in a non-judgmental way.

But what I want us to observe and describe dispassionately are our emotions. Not so much the emotion of anger, but other emotions such as:

- Disappointment
- Frustration
- Sadness
- Feelings of rejection
- Loneliness
- Love
- Lust

So, for example, try to think of the last time you were disappointed. Now if you are not very good at observing and describing your emotions, you may find this quite a difficult task. For sure, all of us get disappointed from time to time and often enough. So, there will be a time in the fairly recent past when you have been disappointed, but can you bring it to mind?

If you can bring it to mind – if you can remember a time when you were recently disappointed – was there any other emotion present? For example, were you angry that somebody had disappointed you? If so, this would be in line with a lot of other people. In fact many people completely short-cut it and, instead of saying they were disappointed with something, they describe themselves as being angry about it. And indeed this is how they immediately feel.

The reason for this is that they have added a layer of judgement to their disappointment so that now they are not only disappointed, they are angry as well. The anger is often referred to as 'the second arrow' (the disappointment being the first arrow). So if we can learn simply to be disappointed, then we can avoid the second arrow thumping into our backs.

So how do we learn just to be disappointed (or whatever) and not angry *and* disappointed? That's where the non-judgemental bit comes on: We simply say to ourselves that we are disappointed and there is an implied 'so what?' tacked on the end. In other words: 'I'm disappointed, but so what – that's life, it's not the first time I've been disappointed and it won't be the last. And I'm one of about six thousand million people who get disappointed from time to time'. So if we can learn to do that (and I can tell you it isn't actually difficult) then we save ourselves the pain of the second arrow – the anger, the whole bad feeling – all of that.

But maybe you said that you can't remember the last time you were disappointed. But can you remember the last time you were angry? I guess you can otherwise you wouldn't be reading the book. If you can, I invite you to think back over that experience and see whether your anger would not have been better described as something else – disappointment, hurt, feeling rejected, etc. If so – and frankly it usually is so – then your anger wasn't really your prime emotion, your anger was the second arrow thumping into your back. You were already hurt or whatever and then you became angry as well, which is more than twice as bad.

So, if this is you, I invite you to look very carefully next time you feel angry and see whether your anger wouldn't be better described as something else. Be generous with yourself – have faith in yourself – allow yourself to say 'yes, actually I'm just very disappointed and hurt' and trust yourself to be able to deal with that because we deal with it in exactly the same way that we did previously, in other words 'actually I'm very disappointed and hurt, but there again it's not the first time I've felt like this and it won't be the last and I'm only one of six thousand million people who get disappointed and hurt from time to time.'

So, in mindfulness terms we are accurately observing and describing our emotions and doing so dispassionately or

non-judgementally. It doesn't much alter the disappointment or hurt, but it does stop the second arrow – the anger.
And this is a massive achievement because it is so often the
second arrow that causes the real problem for us because we
can cope with a certain amount of distress (the first arrow)
but past a certain point we pretty much fail to cope, we go
into a complete meltdown. Most people have experienced
this, so I guess you will know what I'm talking about.

If you want to take it further:

1. Practise accurately describing, observing and describ-
    ing your emotions. Do so non-judgementally, in
    other words simply notice what your emotion is
    and describe it. Don't follow on with anything else
    except maybe to say to yourself, 'So what?!'
2. Try this out a number of times and see if you get
    better at it, and see if it reduces your anger. Frankly,
    I would be surprised if it doesn't; the neatness of the
    strategy and the ease with which one can do it, and
    the enjoyableness of it, all combine together to make
    it an appealing thing to do.
3. You can also spread your mindfulness a bit. For
    example, you can do some mindful eating, just as
    we described with the raisin. But you can apply
    that to everything, you can look carefully at what
    you're about to eat, and once in your mouth you can
    describe to yourself how it feels and tastes, and do so
    in a non-judgemental way.
4. In some ways there is no point to such an exercise,

but it can be quite enjoyable, and it also sets you up nicely to adopt the same approach with your emotions.

5. If you are interested in taking mindfulness further, there are lots of good books about it, and there are one or two good apps for your hand-held device.

18

Strengthening the real you

The ideas I describe in this chapter were prompted by acceptance and commitment therapy (ACT), the work of Steven Hayes, Kirk Strosahl and Kelly Wilson. Acceptance and commitment therapy is so complicated that some people say that if you think you understand it then that just shows how little you understand about it. Well I'm not quite sure I understand it, so maybe that means I'm getting there.

Still there is one clear simple idea that I have grasped, and I think it is a key one for what we are discussing in this book. Do you recollect that in a previous chapter I described how we can get into a state where our normal judgement has been hijacked, we are overtaken by our anger and feel very energised, and very right. You might also remember that I said something similar in an earlier chapter, saying that we normally don't do very well if we simply do what our anger tells us, we are better off doing what our true self tells us to do.

Both of these ideas assume that our 'true self' is well developed, clear and strong – if it isn't then the anger will easily override it. Maybe your true self is good and strong, but I know first-hand that mine certainly benefitted from me working on it, and that is partly what acceptance and commitment therapy is about.

ACT stands for:

Accept your thoughts and feelings and other things out of your personal control.
Commit to a direction in line with your values.
Take action, ACT in line with your values.

And you can see that if you follow these three instructions then this will strengthen up your 'true self' so that it stands a good chance when your anger gets roused. It will be a fair fight between your anger and your true self and hopefully your true self will come out on top.

And we have to be really clear on what our values are, and this is the focus of this chapter. If we can be clear on our values then we can commit to taking action in line with those values. If we don't know what our values are then we are in trouble even before we start.

Why don't you take a moment out to write down what your values are? Just pause for a minute and write your values down somewhere.

There aren't any 'trick questions' in this book although that is about as close as it gets, the reason being that many of us are really very vague about what our values are. If you have totally clear values then congratulations – and I suspect you know that you are in the minority.

So how do we decide upon our values? Russ Harris (who wrote an excellent book called *ACT Made Simple*) said something like the following:

Deep in your heart, what do you want your life to be about? What do you want to stand for? Values describe how we want to behave on an ongoing basis. Clarifying values is an essential step in creating a meaningful life.

It sounds good doesn't it, and it is. But how do we identify our values? Steven Hayes and Russ Harris describe ideas such as these – see if any strike a chord with you:

1. Ask yourself:
   What matters to me overall in life?
   What do I want to stand for?

2. How would you like to see yourself described in an obituary? (Presumably you wouldn't want to see yourself featuring in an obituary at all, but you understand the idea.)

3. More cheerfully, imagine it is your next significant birthday (eighteen, sixty or whatever.) Somebody makes a speech about you, what you stand for, what you mean to them, the role you have played in their life. *In an ideal world*, where you are living your life as you want to, what would you want to hear them say?

4. What do you disapprove of or dislike in the actions of others? How would you act differently, if you were in their shoes? Why?

If you found any of those questions yielded some good answers for you, then I suggest you write them down somewhere, either in a notebook or on the smartphone or computer. The kind of words that I have seen people produce are:

- competent
- integrity
- kind
- responsible
- respect
- dedicated
- enjoys things / is fun
- loyal
- honest
- a team player
- dignified
- collaborative
- empathic / sympathetic
- wise
- secure
- likes learning
- compassionate
- friendly
- generous
- optimistic
- dependable
- flexible

That is a long list, compiled from lots of people and any one person will have a small number of key values, maybe two or three. *Kind and loyal* for example. This doesn't mean that such a person is automatically kind and loyal or naturally kind and loyal; it means that they are committing themselves to taking action in that direction – becoming kind and loyal. This is a long-term day-by-day project and one that is enjoyable and worth doing.

Some people undermine themselves by saying, 'But that's not the way I naturally am' or words to that effect. And it is an important point, even though it does undermine them. We have lots of sections to the brain, one of which pretty much represents what we naturally are. Happily though, most of us want to be more sophisticated than what we naturally are, so as to distinguish us from our ancient ancestors, and I guess that is the kind of reason that inspired you to read this book. We'll talk more about what is going on in the brain, shortly.

So there we are, it is as simple as that. This chapter has been a short one but I think it is at least as important as any. Here we have taken what is sometimes termed a constructional approach in the sense that it is constructing our good side in the sure knowledge that this will stand us in good stead when our anger tries to temporarily take us over. I hope you enjoy the project.

Project

1. Think about your values and, if you wish, discuss your values with other people you know or respect.
2. Notice when you are acting according to your values and (b) notice what it is like to do so.
3. Note down your values – in your smartphone maybe – so you can refer back to them for ever.

Taking it further

The books I mentioned are:

Acceptance and Commitment Therapy by Steven Hayes, Kirk Strosahl and Kelly Wilson (Guilford Press, 1999).

and

ACT Made Simple by Russ Harris (New Harbinger, 2009).

19

Thank goodness for inhibitions

As we have said before, some people view inhibitions as bad things to have. They think in terms of 'being inhibited', equating it with being unexciting and lacking in spontaneity.

In our context the reverse is the case. Remember where the inhibitions box fits into our model (Figure 19.1).

The point here is that anger is an emotion which we may or may not choose to display to other people. So it is possible for somebody to be angry with you without you realising it, simply because they choose not to tell you or not to demonstrate it in any way. And, of course the reverse holds true as well: it is perfectly possible for you to be feeling very irritable and angry and for other people to be totally unaware of it. This is a useful phenomenon and is thanks to our inhibitions. It is no accident that there is an area of the brain whose specific function is to inhibit the expression of every emotion that might occur.

This area of the brain can be damaged temporarily, for example by alcohol, or permanently by injury or some illnesses. Happily, however, it can also be developed. In this chapter we will look at inhibitions, why we want to use them, and how we can develop our ability to use them.

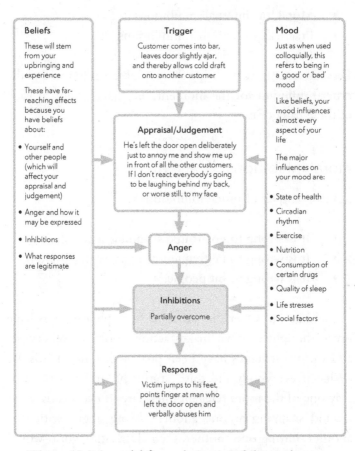

Figure 19.1 A model for analysing irritability and anger

Internal and external inhibitions

Inhibitions fall into two categories:

- Moral, or 'internal' inhibitions.
- Practical, or 'external' inhibitions.

Leaving aside how we bring these inhibitions to mind at the crucial time just for the moment, let's have a look at each of these categories.

Moral inhibitions

Some examples of moral inhibitions are:

- 'It is wrong to go around snapping at people.'
- 'It is wrong to be frequently angry with people.'
- 'It is wrong to hit people.'

. . . and so on. Over thousands of years philosophers have given thought to what makes actions moral or otherwise, and various schemes have been proposed. One such is the 'What if everybody did this?' argument, and this is probably one of the more relevant ones here. If everybody went around snapping at one another, being angry with one another, hitting one another, then clearly the world would be an extremely unrewarding place. Therefore, if it is not okay for everybody to do it, how can it be okay for you or me to do it?

Another basis for morality is the 'adhering to set rules' scheme, of which the Ten Commandments is one example. And this is a powerful constraint on people's behaviour. We all set ourselves rules which control our behaviour – down to the finest detail, sometimes. Some of these rules can be very strange and even abhorrent. For example, there are men who hold to the rule that 'You never hit a woman, unless you're living with her.' Now what possible ethical basis can such a rule have? None that I or the majority of people can see; but even so, this rule governs the behaviour of some men.

Some rules are imposed on us by society and most of us sign up to them. Examples include 'You don't stab people', 'You don't shoot people' and 'You don't hit people'. But of course, not everybody signs up to all of these rules. Most people sign up to the first two of those three, but a significant number do not sign up to the third. I say that simply because some parents still hit their children, although they usually use a euphemism such as 'slap' or 'smack' or 'spank'.

Once you start setting rules for yourself, over and above those that society imposes, then things can get complicated, especially in view of the fact that this should be a simple business. For example, before our children were born, my wife and I set a rule for ourselves that we would never hit them. A good rule, we thought, and indeed we have abided by it. But even this has snags, which I will tell you about.

Just before I do, though, I would like to you to contemplate an incident I witnessed walking through the pedestrian area of a city centre. Nearby, a woman was walking along with her two children of perhaps eight and ten. As they walked along, she was hitting one of them backwards and forwards across the head, saying to him as she did so: 'How many times have I told you not to hit your brother?' The contradictory nature of the mother's words and behaviour somehow produced an almost humorous side to this sorry sight. Nevertheless, the 'give him a taste of his own medicine' thinking that she was demonstrating is common enough. Sadly, however, the all-powerful effect of modelling will probably overwhelm everything else. The young lad will be left with the simple observation that 'it is okay to hit people, even my mother does it'.

But back to my own dilemmas. There we were, smugly bringing up our kids without hitting/smacking/slapping them. And did this mean that they behaved like angels? No, of course it didn't; in fact they behaved just like all other kids. For example, when young, they would shout, squabble, pinch and hit each other. Shout, in particular. So how did I resolve the situation, how did I intervene to stop them shouting and quarrelling? Well, naturally, I shouted louder than either of them.

This usually worked in the short term, but was it a good policy? Clearly not, because I was doing exactly the same as I had seen the woman in the pedestrian area doing: trying to quell a behaviour by exhibiting exactly the same behaviour. So what lesson would my children learn? Presumably 'It's okay to shout, even my father does it'. (You'll be pleased to hear that I didn't do this many times, once the ridiculousness of it had sunk in.)

'Modelling' is the key concept here. This simply refers to the 'model' or 'example' you set. And in the case of parents and children, the example we set is a very powerful one.

Here's another instance of the power of rule-setting. Mo was a young man who had come to see me because he had taken to terminating arguments with his girlfriend by hitting her. The sequence of events seemed to be that they would start arguing, both would start shouting at each other, and the process would only come to an end when he hit her. He then felt terribly guilty, she felt terrible, and this was putting an understandable strain on the whole relationship. And yet, he seemed unable to stop. This was surely strange; one might say, 'If he doesn't want to do it, why doesn't he *stop* doing it?' But, as so often is the case, he seemed to be the victim of his own behaviour. Mo was unable to help himself and so turned to outside help through therapy.

Mo and I talked about his background and he told me about his school and college days (which weren't long ago; he was only in his early twenties at the time). In particular he told me how he seemed to be a natural target for bully-ing. Even in his last year at school a particular fellow student used to pick on him. On one occasion this youth picked on him once too often and, probably accidentally, ripped his shirt. Mo told me how, when this happened, something snapped inside him. Apparently uncontrollably, he just grabbed hold of his tormentor and gave him a thorough pummelling. Unsurprisingly, perhaps, this put an end to the bullying. In fact, not only did the tormentor stop torment-ing Mo, he also seemed to be genuinely remorseful.

Equally unsurprisingly, Mo felt rather pleased with himself; it seemed that he had discovered the answer to many of life's problems, although he did not phrase it consciously and openly to himself in this way. Nevertheless, it was about six months after that incident that he first hit his girlfriend. And from then on there was no turning back; the pattern was established.

So the question is: What rule had Mo established for himself? It seemed to be something like: 'It's okay to hit people, in fact it will solve a lot of problems'.

And yet, when we examine the evidence, this only seemed to be partially true. In the one instance, leaving aside as to whether Mo was 'right' to hit the other guy, it had worked well for him. With his girlfriend, it was working very badly for both of them.

I asked him to try out a new rule, namely: 'It's sometimes okay to get into fights with males my own age, but no one else.' He tried it out, experimentally at first; then, gradually, he 'bought into' the rule and adopted it as his own. On his subsequent appointments he came with his girlfriend, and they told me this new approach was working very well for them. (Incidentally, Mo did *not* then go around getting into fights with males his own age. In fact, he seemed to be naturally a very peaceable kind of character.)

So, we have a first category of inhibitions, the moral category. These inhibitions may be established by the question 'What if everybody went around doing this?' This principle will usually stop us from indiscriminately snapping, shouting and hitting.

The other yardstick for these moral inhibitions is 'obedi-
ence to a rule'. Many rules are the laws of the land and
it's obviously best to go by those. Others, like not hitting
children, we make up for ourselves. Even so, they are very
powerful determinants of our behaviour. I mentioned in
an earlier chapter the man at the bar who stopped himself
being hit by saying to his would-be assailant, 'Hey, I'm
over forty.' By the time the would-be assailant had checked
through his list of rules to see whether there was one which
said, 'You don't hit men over forty' the moment had passed.

Practical inhibitions

The second category of inhibitions is practical; nothing
to do with morality. Inhibitions in this category limit our
behaviour by reminding us of the dire consequences that
might befall us if we don't observe them.

Exercise

Below, I have listed some of the examples we have talked
about in this book, in the form of questions which invite
you to say why the person in question doesn't just do the
very thing that occurs to them. I have filled the first three
in to show you the kind of thing that's in my mind. Have a
go at doing the others.

1. Justin is intensely irritated by his noisy neighbours
   playing their music over-loudly next door to him.

What practical considerations stop him going around and giving his neighbours a real piece of his mind?

Answer: He believes that if he did that, they would probably play their music even louder. And in any case, the guy next door is bigger and fitter than Justin, so he feels he must treat him with some respect.

2. Marius is intensely irritated by his neighbours' kids playing soccer in the street outside and allowing their ball to run all over his garden. What stops him going around and giving the kids and their parents a good telling off?

   Answer: See above. In this case, too, Marius thinks the kids will probably just behave worse, and laugh and jeer at him every time they see him, and the parents might even encourage them to do that.

3. Aisha is intensely irritated by the noise that her husband makes when he is eating. What stops her from jumping up, banging the table and shouting, 'For God's sake why can't you eat like a normal human being?'

   Answer: She's afraid that if she did that it would bring to a head the whole disharmony of the marriage. He would realise that her irritation was not really with his eating, but with him in general, and that his noisy eating symbolises something deeper, to her.

4. Chris, who drives a smart four-wheel drive, is annoyed by the bad driving of a guy in an old wreck.

Chris chases after him and, when the other car has to pause at the next roundabout, feels like driving straight into the back of him. What stops him doing this?

5. Dylan has not got much time for the police so, when he is stopped late one night and asked where he is going and what he is doing, he feels like telling the police officer to mind his own business. In truth, he feels like attacking him. What stops Dylan from doing this?

6. Samantha has a thing about 'bouncers' at the entrance to clubs. So, when a bouncer stops her and her friend from going into a particular club, she screams and shouts at him and launches an apparently energetic attack – but one which, in reality, has no force in it. Why does she not launch a proper full-blooded attack on the bouncer?

Below are what seem to be the answers from the people in question. See how they match up with what you wrote.

4. Chris, who drives a smart four-wheel drive, is annoyed by the bad driving of a character in an old wreck. Chris chases after him and, when the other car has to pause at the next roundabout, feels like driving straight into the back of him. What stops him doing this?

   Answer: He knows that doing so will probably cause a serious accident as a result of which he, Chris, will find himself in court; and the very least that will happen is that he will be banned from driving.

5. Dylan has not got much time for the police so, when he is stopped late one night and asked where he is going and what he is doing, he feels like telling the police officer to mind his own business. In truth, he feels like thumping him. What stops Dylan from doing this?

   Answer: He knows he'll probably end up being arrested and charged, and will lose out in some major way.

6. Samantha has a thing about 'bouncers' at the entrance to clubs. So, when a bouncer stops her and her friend from going into a particular club, she screams and shouts at him and launches an apparently energetic attack – but one which, in reality, has no force in

it. Why does she not launch a proper full-blooded attack on the bouncer?

Answer: She knows she would come off second best, and anyway doesn't want to do anything that could be seen as 'an assault'.

It's clear that these inhibitions have nothing at all to do with 'morality'. They are entirely to do with practical consequences and not wanting to lose out in some way. And none the worse for that.

Summary

In this chapter we have looked at two types of inhibitions: internal and external.

Internal inhibitions are mainly to do with rules we make up for ourselves or other people's rules that we sign up to. It is helpful if we get these rules very clear in our minds – this helps us to abide by them. Some people even write their rules down because it seems to strengthen them.

External inhibitions come from practical considerations about what will happen if you take a particular course of action. These are equally important and equally as 'good' as internal inhibitions.

It is important for us to develop our inhibitions and fine-tune them if we are to manage our anger well.

Project

Try answering the following questions for yourself:

1. What are your internal inhibitions – the rules you have for yourself in regards to anger and irritability?
2. Having read this chapter, is there an additional rule you would like to make for yourself? If so, what is it?
3. How strong are your external inhibitions? (You might judge their strength by asking yourself whether they always manage to control your behaviour in the way you would like them to and, if not, how often they fail to do so.)
4. If you wanted to strengthen your external inhibitions, how might you do so? (We also look at this in the next chapter, but it's also interesting to ponder it now.)

20

So why do we get irritable and angry and what do we do about it?

Following on from the previous chapter, a perfectly reasonable question is: 'If there are so many moral and practical reasons for us to inhibit our irritability and anger, why do we have the capability for anger at all – humans aren't normally designed to feel and do things that have no purpose, so what's the purpose in this case?'

The main answer seems to be that it is a feedback mechanism – a way of letting other people know that what they are doing is going down badly with you. A way, therefore, of people becoming socialised and working together as a society rather than a collection of competing individuals.

In that case, why should we inhibit our inhibition and anger? If it fulfils this useful function of informing people when we feel they are they are 'out of order', presumably if we inhibit it then everything will go haywire. Other people will trample all over us, secure that there is no payback.

And, if taken to extremes, that would be true. If you were never to show any irritation, never to show any anger, this would probably be confusing for people. They wouldn't know when you were pleased and when you were displeased; it would be quite disorientating for those who want to please you.

But there is a happy medium. Some people we know are decidedly 'irritable'. We are not suggesting that they should *never* show any irritation or anger; that would probably be superhuman (and, as we have just noted, not very helpful). There are things in life that *are* irritating, things which prompt a 'normal' person to show some irritation. When we describe a person as 'irritable', however, s/he is going too far, becoming irritated by things that wouldn't irritate a 'normal' person, or getting more irritated than most by slightly irritating things.

So, as ever, it is not a question of 'all or nothing'. Yes, it is sometimes just as well for people to be able to sense that we are irritated or angry. On the other hand, it is very easy to take this much too far, to the point where even the slightest thing irritates us, or where we become irritated if things are not *exactly* as we want them. In that case our irritation and anger mechanism is clearly over-functioning, to the extent that it is counterproductive. When it is functioning at just the right level it provides useful feedback to other people; they can sense when we are slightly irritated and angry with what they are doing and as a result will probably desist. If it is functioning in too extreme a way, those around us get frightened and worried, and our relationships begin to break down.

A good parallel is with jealousy and possessiveness. Most

people rather like their loved ones to exhibit a small amount of jealousy and possessiveness towards them. If this is not the case, many people take it as an indication that they are not really loved. But what happens when this is taken too far? When someone spends all their waking moments worried about what their loved one is doing, whether they are being faithful and loyal? Some people go to the extent of popping home unexpectedly, leaving listening devices around the house or on the phone, even hiring private detectives to follow their loved ones around. Clearly, this level of jealousy and possessiveness is counterproductive and is very quickly going to lead to a breakdown in the relationship.

So, in both instances, whether we are talking about irritability and anger or jealousy and possessiveness, you can have too much of a good thing. In fact, rather like salt, the right amount seems to be very little indeed!

Putting the brakes on

We can see, then, that for all sorts of moral and practical reasons we want to limit our irritability and anger – almost to the extent of stopping it before it gets going. If we keep it down to very low levels it can work extremely well for us and for everybody around us; if we let it get any higher the reverse is the case: it works really badly for us and all around us.

So how do we perform this difficult balancing act, of keeping any irritation and anger down to useful and beneficial levels – down to those very subtle levels where those around us actually feel pleased to see the very occasional irritation from us, simply because it gives them feedback about what is happening?

For a task as complex as this we need a simple analogy. The best I know is that of traffic lights. If you drive around any reasonably large town you will find there is a complex system of interacting traffic lights. For example, near where I live there is a ring road round which I have to drive to get to the motorway. At one point on this ring road there is a particularly distinctive sequence of lights. The first set normally brings you to a halt; for some reason they usually seem to be on red. While you sit waiting at these lights, you can also see that the second set of lights you have to go through is also on red. In due course your first set turns to green, and you move off. If you go off at a very moderate pace, by the time you reach the second set (which is only 40 or 50 metres away) those too are changing to green and you can sail across, although you do have to keep your wits thoroughly about you during this procedure. The same applies to a third set of lights, again only 40 to 50 metres ahead; these too are in sequence with the first and second sets, and you can time things to get across all three in one steady passage.

In summary, what would be a completely unruly flow of traffic is first of all brought to a halt, then allowed to proceed in a thoroughly orderly and controlled fashion. Of course, there are other roads crossing the road I am on, hence the need for lights. An aerial view of this whole procedure would reveal an amazing number of vehicles, all meshing superbly and proceeding at as reasonable a pace as they possibly can. A real feat of interaction and coordination.

Exactly the same happens when two or more people are interacting. Each individual has their own sense of direction, their own pace they want to keep up, their own interests. At the same time they are very keen to mesh with one another, not only because they know that is to their mutual advantage, but also because it's enjoyable and satisfying.

So how does the traffic lights analogy work in practice?

The main thing is to spot a red light! And that's easy. As soon as we see any amount of irritation or anger in us, that is a red light. So we don't just barge across it; that way lies disaster.

When confronted with a red light, irritation and anger in other words, we stop. This is not a 'give way' sign; it is very definitely a 'stop' one. We really have to make sure we come to a complete halt. Sometimes people say 'count to ten'. Well, you can do this if you want; certainly it brings things to a pretty marked stop. On the other hand, you can simply note the presence of the 'red light' (irritability and anger), carry on talking about whatever you like, and then, when the irritability and anger have subsided to a tiny amount (the lights change to amber, if you like) you can get ready to move on to say or do whatever you think is best.

How does that work in practice? Here are some real examples, the first of which – you will not be surprised to learn – concerns Omar, in a draft at the bar.

Omar at the bar

Red light: Yet another man comes in, leaving the door open. Omar experiences a sudden surge of anger, which he recognises as a red light.

Amber light: Quickly, almost instantly, Omar's anger drops to a very low level. Simply refraining from speaking for a moment has helped. He judges the best thing to say.

Green light: Omar leans over towards the man who has just come in and is about to walk past, and says: 'Push the door shut, would you, friend, it leaves a heck of a draft.'

And, moreover, he can repeat this sequence time and again, just as he can manage hundreds of traffic lights on a journey.

Nathaniel dropping mug on floor, irritates Lola

Red light: The sound of the mug smashing on the floor produces a sudden surge in adrenaline in Lola, which she recognises as the red light. She says nothing for an instant, while the anger quickly drops to a more minor level.

Amber light: With her anger at a much lower level, she works out the best response.

Green light: Still with a trace of irritation in her voice, she says: 'Get a brush and sweep that up and put it in the bin, there's a good boy.'

Again, this is an interesting one, because it is not just mugs that Nathaniel breaks; in truth, he is somewhat careless. It is therefore probably appropriate that Lola's voice has just a dash of irritation in it. It's certainly very genuine, she really feels the irritation. But by thinking in terms of the traffic lights procedure she puts it into a useful context rather than a destructive one.

Vicky tells of Danny and her underwear

Red light: Danny felt intensely angry that Vicky had broken a very intimate confidence, not just to a few other people, but on the radio. This intense anger persisted for several days. He therefore said nothing.

Amber light: When the anger had subsided to a more manageable level, Danny worked out the best way to approach the subject.

Green light: At a moment when there was plenty of time, and he and Vicky were getting on reasonably well, he said: 'I'll tell you something I think we should talk about, because you know I was really angry about what you said on the radio the other day. It seems to me we should talk about what needs to be kept between the two of us and what can be said to others, because I know both of us come under pressure from smart interviewers to say things we'd rather not. So I guess we ought to get our act together now about how we're going to cope with that.'

The traffic lights technique is a remarkably strong and powerful one. But there are several points to be made.

Sometimes the 'red light' stays on for a very short period of time, barely a second or two. Omar in the bar, and Lola with Nathaniel who drops the mug on the floor, are examples of this. In other cases the red light stays on for hours or even days – as with Danny and Vicky.

Secondly, you don't always get what you want. Amy is an example of this. She never got to the point where her daughter set about happily tidying her bedroom all on her own. And we have to recognise that there's no law that says we should get what we want, any more than other people always get what they want. There's no need to 'awfulise' this phenomenon. It's just the way things are.

The third point, and the best news, is that just as we get good at coping with real traffic lights, we also get good at coping with these metaphorical ones. So, whereas previously Omar became more and more incensed every time somebody left the door to the bar open, he now became more and more skilled at going through the traffic lights procedure. So each time he said, 'Push the door to, would you, friend, it leaves a heck of a draft', it seemed like the first time he had said it, as far as the hearer was concerned; but in fact, this was now a skilled procedure he had developed.

Likewise, and perhaps in particular, for Lola with Nathaniel the mug-breaker. Nathaniel gave Lola plenty of practice in spotting red lights, but Lola did her bit by recognising them and moving through them efficiently and productively.

Exercise

- Think of a 'red light' that has occurred over the last two days: something that actually made you angry, or potentially could have done.
- Did you recognise it as any sort of a red light and stop at that point?
- Did you stop and wait for the anger to subside to a very small amount and then decide on your best way forward? Did you then move off along the productive path you'd chosen?

Well, unless you've read this book before, presumably you've answered no to one or more of those questions. So here is another . . .

Exercise

- Again, what exactly was the 'red light'? In other words, what happened to make you angry?
- What would 'stopping' have meant in that situation? In other words, could you simply have said nothing, or would that have looked strange? Would you perhaps have had to carry on talking in some way or carry on doing what you were doing? In that case the 'red light' is simply not responding to your anger but instead carrying on with what you were doing.
- When your anger has subsided to a low level, what would have been the best path to take? This is the

amber phase: your anger is at a low level, and you (not your anger) are deciding on the best way forward.

- What exactly would 'green' have looked like? In other words, what would you have said or done? What tone of voice would you have used?

If this all sounds very complicated, that's misleading. It is a very simple and very enjoyable procedure. It is best, however, to go through it in your mind a few times, just as the second of these two exercises suggests. Each time you hit 'red', recognise it as such, allow the anger to subside to a very low level, and then decide on your best way forward. Then move forward, actually do what you've decided on (green).

Tip

There is only one trap in this procedure, and that is to kid yourself that you're at amber when in fact you're still on red. Remember, the characteristic of being at amber is that your irritation and anger are at very low levels. Sometimes, it is true, this may be just half a second after the intense initial burst of anger. At other times, however, it is a good while afterwards.

Summary

In this chapter we have looked at:

- Why we get irritable and angry: the idea that a very low level of irritability and anger provides useful feedback to those around us, while anything above this very low level is counter-productive and simply puts everybody on edge.
- How we can bring inhibitions to mind when we want them, and act on them usefully by using the traffic lights procedure.

Project

Two projects come out of this chapter:

1. The practical project is the traffic lights one. Really practise spotting 'red lights'. In other words, practise spotting when you become angry. Allow it to sink to a low level (amber) as quickly as possible. Only at that point do you decide what would be a reasonable way forward. Then, when you've decided, move on to green; in other words, put into practice what you think

is the best way forward. And remember, you can't always have your own way!

2. As ever, review your successes, either mentally or on paper. It's good to analyse successes because it shows us the route to success.

21

The bottom line: response

You know what they mean by 'the bottom line'? It comes from business and refers to the bottom line of the accounts: the final profit (or loss) figure. It doesn't matter whether the head of the business has been extremely hard-working and everyone else in the firm incredibly conscientious; if the bottom line is that the business made a loss then that, in a sense, is all that matters. Conversely, it doesn't matter that another business might have a lazy and lethargic head and an opportunistic workforce; if the bottom line is that they are making a healthy profit, then that, in a sense, is all that matters.

It's the same here. In our model (Figure 21.1) we are now looking at the 'response' box. The point is that if our final response is an acceptable one (i.e. non-irritable, non-angry) then it really doesn't matter what our beliefs are, what our mood is, what triggered things off, how angry we got, how good we are at implementing inhibitions, and so on. In theory at any rate, you can have everything piling up against you and still make an acceptable response. And in fact it's not just theory; it can and does happen in practice too.

So, if you are looking for a short cut, this is it although, if I were you, I'd regard it as the final piece of the jigsaw; that way you have everything pulling on your side.

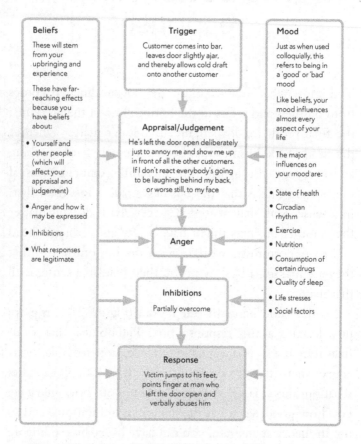

Figure 21.1 A model for analysing irritability and anger

Either way, as far as anybody else is concerned all they can see is your response. It doesn't matter to them what's been going on inside your head; if you respond irritably and angrily then you are an irritable and angry person. Equally, if you respond in a non-irritable and a non-angry way, then that is how you are defined.

So, given that most of us would prefer *not* to be seen as irritable and angry, what do we do? The good news here is that we have covered most of what we need to cover already. The three key concepts are:

- The traffic lights analogy.
- Modelling yourself on a good example.
- Reviewing successful (and unsuccessful) incidents.

Traffic lights

Let's go through the traffic lights analogy first.

The 'red light' comes on when you can see that you are about to make an irritable and angry response – or at least, a response that will be seen by other people as irritable or angry. You treat this impulse as a red light: in other words, you literally stop. All you do is *not* say or do whatever it is you were going to say or do. If other, similar, things come into your mind, then you stay at the stop light. You get ready to move off *only* when you start thinking of alternative, non-irritable, non-angry responses.

Sometimes you can only think of one 'reasonable' response. Sometimes it takes a long time for such a response to occur to you. In that case, it simply means you are stuck on red for a long time. This is, of course, entirely true to life; just occasionally you come across lights which seem to be stuck on red for ever. But eventually, sometimes after half a second, sometimes after half a week, you think of a reasonable response. That is your cue to move on to green. The 'green light' is simply doing whatever the reasonable response is. But remember, 'reasonable' is in *your* judgement, not the judgement of your anger. You know full well that your anger tells you to do things that the genuine *you* would disagree with. So, don't let your anger have the last word; insist that *you* do.

One of the examples we used earlier was Lola coping with her careless son Nathaniel, who's prone to dropping and breaking things – mugs, for example. She describes one instance where, as soon as the mug smashed on the floor, she felt an overwhelming surge of anger; she just wanted to shout anything at him. She also describes recognising that as a red light, and simply keeping her mouth shut for a moment. This was, more or less, a 'half-second' red light. No sooner had she come screeching to a halt on red than she quickly saw that all she needed to do was to get him to sweep it up. In other words, she moved straight on to amber, where a reasonable response occurred to her; and then on to green: 'Just sweep it up, there's a good boy,' said with the merest hint of annoyance.

The same with Chris, the character who was prone to road rage. He trained himself to recognise the red light, too. He described an instance where somebody pulled in front of him rather more sharply than he felt they should have done; having braked, he literally felt his foot having a will of its own, wanting to get on to the accelerator to 'tailgate' the offender. He had by this stage of training learnt to recognise this impulse and he simply refrained from giving into it. The 'right response' for Chris was telling himself to 'drive by his own standards'. The green light was simply doing that: taking his instruction literally, driving well and responsibly.

Following a good example

The second concept is that of modelling yourself on a good example. This is also is one of my favourites. The great thing about having an example to model yourself on is that you can clearly envisage what responses you can make. All you have to do is to ask yourself: 'What would he or she do in this situation?' and you have a ready-made template for your own behaviour. Then it's just a case of mimicking it.

So, by spending a couple of minutes now, you can save yourself endless hours of difficulty later on. All you need to do in that brief time is to think of somebody who would make a really good example for you. Here are a few tips to help you choose:

- You are looking for somebody, preferably the same gender as you but not necessarily, who typically makes non-irritable and non-angry responses. Someone who is difficult to get angry. Do *not* model yourself on somebody who easily becomes irritable and angry!

- It should be a person who you like, even admire; someone you would be pleased to be thought similar to.
- The individual you're modelling yourself on does not have to be 'perfect'. They may have elements to them that you would not want to copy. Even so, by and large, you like or admire them and, certainly, they are non-irritable and non-angry.
- The person you bring to mind may be someone you know from real life, or someone you know only in a public role, perhaps from television or radio. It is important, however, that you have a very vivid idea of what they say and do, so that you can copy it easily.

You might find more than one person to model yourself on. This is not necessarily a good thing, because in the heat of the moment you need to have one clear image to copy. So you're probably best off, certainly in the initial stages, having just one person to bring instantly to mind, so that you can quickly ask yourself what he or she would do in this situation.

Hence Lemy (the one whose wife, Ella, irritated him by laughing and joking with other men) used Jamie as a model. (Jamie's wife, Michelle, was also a touch flirtatious, but only in the same harmless way as Ella.) This was a highly appropriate model for Lemy because he knew both Jamie and Michelle well, recognised that Michelle had many similarities to Ella, and could see that if only he could bring himself to behave like Jamie, then all would be well. In fact this worked out especially well because it meant that the four of them got on better than before, with each of the quartet involved effectively in 'mirroring' one another.

Aaron, the father of the twelve-year-old boy who hadn't done his homework, used the character of a middle-aged teacher from a television soap opera as his model. This was an interesting one; I wasn't convinced this was a very good role model to choose: first because this character was rather older than Aaron and second because he was in fact a teacher and was therefore in a position to help youngsters with homework quite readily. Aaron wasn't particularly good at his son's homework himself, so wasn't that good at helping. The third thing that slightly worried me was that this character was a bit 'too good to be true', so I was worried that Aaron might be setting himself an impossible target. Happily I was proved wrong, and Aaron found his role model a very good one. Even when he couldn't help his son, Marius, it still seemed to carry him through. Such is the power of 'modelling'.

Reviewing

You will recognise that this idea comes up time and again. Quite rightly too; it is very important indeed. This is how we really consolidate things: by reviewing both good and bad events, and taking our lessons from them.

So, if you do let yourself down at all (i.e. get too irritable and too angry) then, as soon as you have got back to your normal self, undertake a thorough review. What would you have preferred to do in that situation? (In other words, what response would you have preferred to make?) Would it have been best to use the traffic lights technique, the modelling technique, or to combine the two? When you combine the two you simply stop at the red light of irritability and anger, think of your role model to help you come up with a suitable response (the amber light), and then move off to mimic that response (the green light).

So you literally relive the situation, but give it a better ending. This, technically, is known as 'cognitive rehearsal'. It is very effective because, as mentioned before, the brain doesn't mind much whether you're doing things in reality or in imagination. So you are treading the path through the jungle, preparing a path so that the next time a similar situation arises you're more likely to respond in the way you want rather than in the way your habit or your anger tells you.

A note of caution

There is one trap in reviewing, and that is that you simply relive whatever it is that made you angry. Be careful to skirt around this trap. The whole point of reviewing is to 'relive' a better response. Certainly people do and say things which we would prefer they didn't do and say, but that does not mean we have to respond badly. So, we relive and practise (mentally) the response we'd prefer to make.

Just as important, possibly even more so, is to relive our successes. When we see something happen that would formerly have produced a really bad response from us, and yet, this time, we handle it well, we must take time to indulge in self-congratulation. As soon as possible after the event, do a review in just the same way as if you had *not* responded as you would have wished. Again, take care to walk round the trap of simply reviewing what might have made you angry. Rather, review how you managed to respond as well as you did. You can even take it a step further and imagine various other triggers and how you would respond to them in a non-irritable, non-angry way.

Summary

- In this chapter we have seen that we could, if we wished, cut through everything else to the 'bottom line': how we respond. No matter what triggers are put in our way, we are responsible for our own responses.
- There are three good ways for you to get yourself to produce the kind of responses you want to, and those three ways mesh with each other.
- First is the traffic lights technique. When you feel a surge of irritability and anger you simply stop. And you stay on 'red' until you can think of a reasonable response (from you rather than

your anger); this is 'amber'. Once you've got that response clearly in mind you can move on to 'green' and implement it.

- Second is the technique of modelling yourself on a good example. You think of a particular person who always (so far as you know) responds well in adversity, in other words in a non-irritable, non-angry way. You hold this person in mind constantly and, when you are confronted with potential irritability- and anger-producing situations, you respond as s/he would do. Eventually this becomes part of you: you will have grafted these better responses on to the good elements of your own personality.

- Third is the technique of reviewing: instances where you responded badly and – especially – those where you responded well. In both cases you rehearse future responses where you literally envisage the potentially anger-producing stimulus (but avoid the trap of getting involved in reliving it) and rehearse the response you would prefer to make.

Project

Two good things to do:

- Start with the traffic lights technique. Become razor-sharp at recognising approaching irritability and anger, and put yourself on red straight away. Think of the person you have set as an example to model yourself on, and what s/he would do in this situation. This puts you on to amber, because you now have a picture of a really good (non-irritable, non-angry) response. Then move on to green; in other words, implement that response convincingly and with enthusiasm.
- Review the times you successfully handle potentially anger-provoking situations, analyse how you did it, give yourself a pat on the back. If you want, also review the times when you respond badly and what you should have done instead. Both of these are good things to do.

This is a very solid project which will be of tremendous benefit to you if you put your heart into it.

22

What's happening in the brain when we get angry

In this chapter I want us to look in greater depth at what is happening in the brain when we get angry. We have briefly described it in chapter 1, and now I want to look at it further, and especially look at what we can do to control the 'instant anger' the primitive parts of the brain can produce. It is relevant to understanding our anger and irritability and especially the conundrum whereby we seem to do things we don't want to do. 'Whatever was I thinking?' and similar statements of bewilderment are common enough when you talk to angry and irritable people.

The limbic system

The limbic system is pretty much the key to understanding things. The word limbic comes from the Latin for peripheral, so has nothing to do with arms and legs in this case but is simply the term which was given to a chunk of brain which appeared to be peripheral to the main body of brain. It is where the amygdala and hypothalamus are housed and is largely responsible for our emotions. Carl Sagan sometimes refers to it as the reptilian brain, Paul Gilbert often refers to it as the (evolutionarily) old brain, and I quite like to refer to it as the primitive brain. All of these terms probably get across the idea that you find this part of the brain in most mammals; it is responsible for many of our emotions, drives and instincts.

Because it houses the amygdala (Latin for almond – it is an almond-sized, almond-shaped structure responsible for much of our emotion), when we get overcome with anger or other strong emotion it is sometimes referred to as 'an amygdala hijack' because it is as though our capacity for rational thought has indeed been hijacked. People also refer to this state as 'the red mist having descended on them' or being 'besides themselves'. Some countries even recognise this in law where they have a category of crime referred to as 'crimes of passion', implying that the person was so 'hijacked' by their emotions at the time that they temporarily lacked compos mentis – or sufficient equanimity to have reasonable judgement.

The cerebral cortex

This is the part of the brain that strives to make us more civilised than the limbic system would naturally have us be. It is responsible for thinking, planning, inhibitions, movement, understanding the images that the eyes collect and the sounds that the ears hear, and so on. It is what we normally think of as the brain, especially for example when we might describe somebody as 'cerebral' meaning that they may spend a lot of time on crosswords, logical puzzles, thinking deeply about and discussing matters.

The interaction between the limbic system and the cerebral cortex

This is where things get interesting. I think it was Carl Sagan who pointed out the unfortunateness of us are designed with one part of the brain that can lust after controlling the world and another part of the brain that can work out how we might achieve that. Adolf Hitler springs to mind, but he is only one of a number.

Equally I remember seeing someone who was apparently unable to prevent himself from attacking and sexually assaulting small boys. Such was the drive coming from his limbic system that he simply couldn't resist doing this. His thinking brain – the cerebral cortex – eventually reached the decision that the only way out was to kill himself and he took action in line with this. (In fact he was 'rescued' by a surprise visitor to his house so he survived, spending the rest of his life in prison.) This is an extreme case, but it does illustrate the power of the drive coming from the primitive brain.

In defence of the primitive brain I should also point out that it is responsible for producing the emotions and drives that generate the brave and altruistic behaviour we see on a daily basis. People leaving their comfortable homes to risk their lives by travelling to help people in countries suffering from an epidemic of a deadly virus, for example. In the terms of the cerebral cortex such behaviour 'makes no sense', it is driven by something much deeper inside us.

Marsha Linehan has produced a diagram which maybe has a basis in what we're talking about here. She describes the rational mind and the emotional mind and draws them as two overlapping circles, where the overlapping portion is referred to as 'the wise mind' taking account of both rationality and emotion. The idea is that we can act from the wise mind, again taking account of both parts of the brain. This seems like an excellent idea and is surely what happens for example in 'chair work' – see Chapter 13 on that.

But one of the problems we have with anger and irritability is that the primitive brain operates so much more quickly than the rational brain. So, we are sometimes angry even before the thinking brain has thought out whether we are entitled to be so. This causes problems for us. Things can happen that make us instantly angry, our reaction will be equally instant and, often enough we will regret it. This is where the comments such as 'whatever was I thinking' come in. And in reality of course we weren't thinking, that is the whole point – our reaction came from the primitive brain not the rational, thinking brain.

So what can we do about it? By its nature it is not something we can rationally think through and plan how to react against because it comes from the primitive brain. On the other hand we know full well that the primitive brain is sometimes more irritable and sometimes more easily aroused to anger than at other times.

If you keep a diary of the sort we described earlier then you may be able to analyse and detect some pattern; to see when your primitive brain is most easily aroused to anger. If you don't, I would suggest that certain things may make you more susceptible, such as:

- Being ill or in pain
- Being tired
- Being hungry
- Being intoxicated
- Being unfit or not having had any recent exercise
- Being worried
- Being depressed
- Certain people or situations

So the least we can do is to recognise these things. And to minimise the number of times we are tired, hungry, intoxicated, unfit, worried or depressed.

'Certain people or situations' is an interesting category though. You may have grasped that anger and irritability are subjects of personal relevance to me and I'm proud to say I have conquered them. Or, at least, as much as any of us do. Still, I was at a lunch table of six people recently and the woman next to me was irritating me so much that I had to make an excuse to change places. I would argue this was the right thing to do rather than to sit there struggling to control my irritability. In fact the best way of completely eliminating it was to move to a different place on the table. I think this is a perfectly good strategy and I would urge you to do the same if ever it is necessary or you find yourself in a parallel situation.

What about 'certain situations'. One category of certain situations for me is art galleries. I can't stand them. This is unfortunate as my wife has a postgraduate degree in the history of art and just loves them. (Just in case you spring to the conclusion that the reason I don't like them is because my wife does like them, I don't think that's true: I like lots of things that my wife likes.) With just two exceptions (the National Portrait Gallery in London and the Metropolitan Museum in New York, if you're interested) every other art gallery I've been to puts me into a state of gloomy irritability. I have no idea why, maybe I was dragged round such places as a child and have ever since associated them with torment, who knows. What I do know is that I'm well advised to avoid them, which is just what I do, and again, to me this is not cheating; it is common sense, and a course of action I commend to you if you can identify any parallels in your own life. (Incidentally, my wife adopts the same strategy with car showrooms, which bore her.)

Taking it further

If you want to see a humorous example of the primitive brain in action, search for 'Ellen scares Taylor Swift' on YouTube. As the title suggests, Ellen DeGeneres springs out on Taylor Swift who instantly collapses to the floor in fright. You can see her rational brain slowly regaining control but you can also see that her primitive brain had immediately put her into emergency mode, a mode which she comes out of more slowly than she went into, and seeks comfort to achieve.

I listed some factors that might 'inflame' the primitive brain. Are any of them relevant to you? If so tick them off and make a plan of action. Are there any others you would add to the list? Here they are again:

- Being ill or in pain
- Being tired
- Being hungry
- Being intoxicated
- Being unfit or not having had any recent exercise.
- Being worried
- Being depressed
- Certain people or situations

If you are interested, you might like to google images of the brain to see what it actually looks like and see if you can spot the parts we have discussed.

23

'But I'm not always irritable, just sometimes': mood

The bad news about this chapter is that it is long. But there are two bits of good news: the first is that the subject matter is naturally interesting and relevant. The second is that there are clear subheads so you can pick and choose the bits you think are going to be *most* interesting and relevant for you personally, if you'd prefer to.

Do you ever have that experience where you just *feel* irritable? No one has even done anything yet, but you know that if they did then it would really irritate you. Or you are with other people and absolutely everything anybody says or does, and the way they do it, irritates you.

Perhaps other people don't realise you're feeling that way, perhaps you're able to keep it to yourself – possibly as a result of reading the previous chapter on 'responses'. But inside you're just feeling 'prickly'.

Colloquially, this is referred to as 'being in a bad mood', and this about sums it up. Technically, too, that feeling

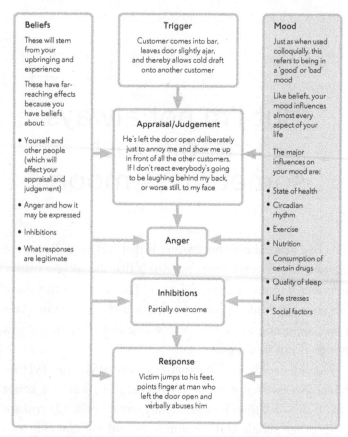

Figure 23.1 A model for analysing irritability and anger

comes under the heading of 'mood'. Back in Part One we looked at the kind of things that influence mood, namely: routine, exercise, nutrition, drugs, sleep, illness, stress and social factors (as above). If we can get these factors right, then we are much less likely to find ourselves in 'a bad mood'.

Interestingly, many people have got so many of these factors awry that they spend a good deal of their lives in a bad mood, and indeed feel that this is 'part of life'. The good news is that this is not so; it's perfectly possible – and reasonably easy – to sort out these factors so that recurrent 'bad moods' become past history.

So, let's take them in turn.

Routine

The body loves routine, doing the same things at the same time most days. Don't be tricked by the idea that 'routine' need be boring. On the contrary, you can if you wish lead the most exciting life of anybody in the world; just make sure you do it every day!

The two *main* things that the body wants to do at regular times are eating and sleeping. Of the two, sleeping is probably the more important. So what you need to do is to go to bed and get up at roughly the same time most days.

Likewise, you need to try to eat at roughly the same times most days. The best way of doing this is to set yourself times for breakfast, lunch, tea and supper (if those are the meals you eat), and then give yourself half an hour's leeway either way. So, you might say that you eat breakfast at 8 a.m., lunch at 1 p.m., tea or snack at 5 p.m. and supper at 8 p.m., which would in fact mean that you had breakfast some time between 7.30 a.m. and 8.30 a.m., lunch at some time between 12.30 p.m. and 1.30 p.m., tea or a snack at some time between 4.30 p.m. and

5.30 p.m., and supper at some time between 7.30 p.m. and 8.30 p.m.

I labour the point because I have seen some people who become over-meticulous about eating at *exactly* the same time every day, and that can be constricting and difficult to maintain. All I am suggesting is that you eat and sleep at *roughly* the same times, most days.

And what happens if you don't? If you know what jet lag is like, then that's what your life becomes, except that you are permanently in a state akin to jet lag. There is nothing mystical about how jet lag occurs: it has nothing to do with jet engines or aeroplanes in themselves; it is simply that one moves from one time zone to another, and this upsets the 'body clock', one's physical rhythm or routine.

Technically, this is known as the 'circadian rhythm' – the rhythm of regularity around a 24-hour cycle that the body likes to maintain.

And when you're in a state of jet lag – which is often characterised as 'tired and irritable' – you are, sure enough, irritable. So, just by ensuring that you maintain a regular routine you may massively reduce your irritability.

This all leads to a very clear and powerful project to get into a routine.

Step 1: List all of the following:

- Get-up time:
- First meal time:

- Second meal time:
- Third meal time:
- Fourth meal time (if any):
- Bedtime:

Step 2: Stick to the times you have written, within 30 minutes either way.

Step 3: You can make a diary of this if you want; in other words, simply record the actual times you eat and sleep. You might be surprised how difficult it is to keep them regular, especially if you're not in the habit of doing so. However, persist; this is one of the linchpins in producing a stable mood for yourself.

Taking exercise

Yes, I know you've heard it before, that exercise is good for you. Well, I'm afraid it's entirely true: human beings are indeed designed to take exercise. It lifts the mood, strengthens up all manner of physical factors, and is generally absolute magic.

The only good news (if you are anything like me) is that exercise does not have to be strenuous. You do not necessarily have to go to a gym and 'work out'. Walking is just as effective.

Conventional wisdom says that aerobic exercise is best, but more recent research seems to suggest that any exercise is good exercise. So, walk whenever you can, run upstairs – generally just get as much exercise as you possibly can fit in. If you want to go swimming as well, or join a gym, or take up yoga or pilates, then of course this is excellent too. But don't do any strenuous exercise without checking things out with your doctor.

A couple of tips

Three factors that have cropped up fairly regularly with people I have seen are as follows:

- People (especially, but not only, women) say that they would walk but they are inhibited from doing so by the wrong shoes. We are not talking about 'serious' walking; just walking to and from the bus stop, or even upstairs some-times. Clearly there is a question of how much priority is being given to exercising here; give it a bit more priority and make sure you have shoes that are comfortable enough to walk in and, if you like, even look good as well.
- Some people, whose natural opportunities for exercise are virtually nil, say that when they get home they are too tired to exercise. Ironically,

if they could make themselves exercise, then the exercise itself would make them feel more energetic. The second way of looking at it (because it is in fact very difficult to 'make' yourself exercise) is again that they should give the exercise more priority: in other words, exercise earlier in the morning, at midday, or at some other time, if they know that they are going to be too tired in the evening. (And, in turn, this would also make them feel less tired in the evening.)

- Some people are tempted to mix exercise with anxiety. For example, I saw one man who deliberately set off slightly late to catch the bus every morning. This meant that he would have to walk fairly briskly down the road to the bus stop. This is a pity; exercise is meant to be a natural and anxiety-free activity!

Exercise project

This too is a key area with massive potential benefits for you.

- The best project is simply to keep a diary of how much exercise you get. This can be 'endemic' exercise, where exercises are simply 'built into your routine' by way of walking from one place to another and so forth. In fact, to make it part and parcel of your routine is probably a very good idea; this means it won't slip once your enthusiasm wanes! Or it can be 'scheduled' exercise: deliberately going for a walk, or for a swim, or for a session in the gym.

- Either way, it is a very good idea to record how much exercise you're getting; indeed it can be interesting – and salutary – to see just how little one sometimes gets!

The final question is: just how much exercise should you get? The answer is: pretty well as much as you like. For those of us in a 'normal' routine it is difficult to get much exercise. Just make sure you get plenty of non-strenuous activity. To be breathing faster than normal, and possibly even sweating, is a good thing; to be noticeably breathless and in discomfort may not be.

Nutrition

In most of the Western world people certainly consume plenty of calories. But whether you get a diet that is good for you is perhaps another matter.

There often seems to be a lot of conflicting information around about what constitutes a good diet, and that sometimes means that people feel like giving up and eating whatever they feel like. That is a pity, because it is simple enough to get a reasonably balanced diet.

Current conventional wisdom is best summarised by saying there are four main types of foods:

1. Fruit and vegetables.
2. High-carbohydrate foods such as bread, rice, potatoes, pasta.
3. High-protein foods such as meat, fish, poultry.
4. High-fat foods such as oily fish, avocadoes, eggs, milk, nuts, etc.

. . . and that we should eat them all. There is nothing 'wrong' with any of the four categories; it's simply a matter of proportion.

It is probably a mistake to actively avoid particular types of food unless you have a clearly diagnosed allergy to them – as in the case, for some people, of nuts. For instance, it can be unwise to actively avoid cholesterol, because excessively low levels of cholesterol have been shown to be associated with low mood. (But, equally, taking a moderate amount of cholesterol does *not* necessarily mean eating a lot of biscuits and chocolates; some of the best forms of cholesterol occur in oily fish such as mackerel, herring, etc.) Similarly, being short of any of the categories has been shown to have an adverse effect.

The next thing is: how good are you at digesting your food? No doubt you were told as a youngster that you need to chew your food properly before swallowing – and it's still true! The reason for this is not only that digestive juices are secreted in the mouth, but that chewing also stimulates the production of other juices in the digestive tract, so that, when the food arrives there, it is 'expected'.

It is best if you can 'put your mind to' eating, rather than eating while you are on the move, talking in too involved a way with other people, and so forth. And it's generally thought to be good to eat unprocessed food as far as possible because that way you can better get a sense of what food your system wants at any particular time.

And finally, it is still true that some people don't drink enough water. And it *is* probably best to say 'water' rather than 'fluids', even though the latter sounds so much more technical! The trouble is that if you think in terms of 'fluids' it opens the door to too much coffee, tea, fruit juice, fizzy drinks etc. Best to think in terms of water. You don't have to drink any more than you want, but do drink enough.

Nutrition project

There's no need to go overboard on this one. Just ensure the following:

- Eat an approximately balanced diet, as described above.

- Give your body a good chance to properly digest the food you eat by having some respect for mealtimes, food and your digestive tract! Remember, it is not so much the case that 'we are what we eat' as 'we are what we properly digest'.
- Drink enough water.

I say 'there's no need to go overboard' simply because I wouldn't want you to get obsessed with what you eat, how you eat it and what you drink with it. Nevertheless, nutrition is important; so, if it's especially relevant to you, make sure you sort it out. Personally I've found it to have a huge effect.

Caffeine

Caffeine is an offender as far as disrupting mood is concerned, so let's have a look where it comes from. The table overleaf shows us that the major sources of caffeine are coffee (including instant), tea (more or less on a par with instant coffee, which surprises many people), energy drinks and cola drinks. There is also a fair amount in dark chocolate, especially if you eat lots of it!

TABLE: THE CAFFEINE CONTENT OF SOME DRINKS AND FOODS:

Item	Average caffeine content (mg)
Coffee (5oz/140g cup)	
brewed drip method	115
brewed percolator	80
instant	65
decaffeinated, brewed	3
decaffeinated, instant	2
Tea	
brewed (5oz/140g cup)	50
instant (5oz/140g cup)	30
iced (12oz/340g glass)	70
Cocoa beverage (5oz/140g cup)	4
Chocolate milk beverage (8oz/227g)	5
Milk chocolate (1oz/28g)	6
Dark chocolate, semi-sweet (1oz/28g)	20

Coca-Cola (12oz/340g)	45.6
Diet Coke (12oz/340g)	45.6
Pepsi Cola (12oz/340g)	38.4
Diet Pepsi (12oz/340g)	36
Pepsi Light (12oz/340g)	36

It comes as a surprise to some people that caffeine can have the far-reaching effects it does. It has been shown to be associated with irritability and is known for its sleep-disturbance properties and the 'jittery' effect that many people have when they drink too much.

In summary, caffeine is one of those substances that is best taken strictly in moderation. There is some evidence that at such a level (around three cups of instant coffee per day) it has quite a good anti-depressant effect; any more and you might need to look at cutting down, back to around that daily level of three cups.

If you are drinking an excessive amount of coffee (and I've come across people who drink thirty cups a day), the best way of cutting down is first of all to halve your current consumption. Then hold that level steady for a week or two. Then halve it again. Then hold that level for a week or two, and halve it again if necessary – keeping going until you get to around three cups a day.

You may well find it surprisingly difficult to cut back because, although most people don't think they are addicted to the amount of caffeine they consume, you may well be. Common withdrawal symptoms include painful headaches and tiredness, although in total it appears that caffeine depletes your energy levels rather than boosts them. Some people who have headaches first thing in the morning or at weekends find that they are associated with caffeine withdrawal because, naturally enough, one doesn't normally consume caffeine through the night and many people drink a lot more caffeine during the working week than at weekends.

In summary, then, limit yourself to around three cups of instant coffee or its equivalent each day. And even then, don't have one of those in the evening time or it will probably interfere with your sleep. Caffeine has a 'half-life' of around six hours, so if you have a cup of coffee at 2 p.m. it will be 8 p.m. before it has diminished to half its original effect, and even at 2 a.m. it will still have a quarter of its effect.

Alcohol

Pretty much the same applies to alcohol. In moderation it's fine, but in excess it really is troublesome.

The recommended weekly maximum in the UK is 14 units. This is 350 mls of 40% spirits, 1 litre (one and a third bottles) of typical 14% wine, or 2.8 litres (slightly under 5 pints) of 5% beer.

Current US recommendations are for a slightly lower intake; the Connecticut Clearinghouse ('a program of Wheeler Clinic Inc., funded by the Department of Mental

Health and Addictions Service') says that 'moderate drinking' should not be exceeded, and defines 'moderate' intake as one drink a day for females and two drinks a day for males, where one drink is equivalent to 1.5 ounces of distilled spirit (40% alcohol by volume), 5 ounces of wine or 12 ounces of regular beer.

I expect that the UK maxima will be lowered in due course. Anyway, if you drink much more than this and also find yourself troubled by irritability, then you really need to work hard at getting down to these limits as a maximum.

The real problem with alcohol is that it interferes with your sleep. Contrary to popular belief, the chances are that your quality of sleep is actually impaired rather than improved by consuming alcohol. Obviously, taken in large amounts it leaves you hungover, and taken even in not very great amounts it still leaves you under par the next day.

Alcohol project

- This one is clear and simple: get down to the recommended maximum of alcohol per week.
- Obviously this is an important one, not only because of the implications for your irritability, but also in terms of minimising the damage alcohol does to your liver and brain in particular.

- If you can manage this by yourself, simply by starting up a new habit of drinking less, then so much the better. If you need some outside help, it's worth getting it. Your family doctor might be able to recommend somebody, or you can get in touch with Alcoholics Anonymous (local contact numbers are in the phone book); you don't have to be drinking as much as you think in order to get help from them. Also, and importantly, a lot of people find all the help they need and more from self-help books.

Recreational ('street') drugs

This category covers a great many drugs, some of which may have interactions with one another, so I don't propose to say too much here. I would rather leave it to your own judgement. Given what we have said above about the 'routine' drugs of caffeine and alcohol and the damaging effects that they have been shown to have on us, you can probably judge for yourself what effect other drugs might be having on you, if you are taking any, and what you had best do about it!

Smoking

Some researchers claim that smoking reduces irritability and anger whereas others refute this saying that the effect only holds good for smokers – in other words, if a smoker is craving a smoke he or she is more likely to be irritable or angry and this effect is reduced if they have a smoke, whereas simply feeding cigarettes to non-smokers (or people who have given up smoking) doesn't reduce their proneness to irritability and anger. In any event, the health risks associated with smoking mean that there can only be one piece of advice, and everybody knows what that is.

Sleep

The importance of sleep is very difficult to overstate. If you can get into the routine of having a good night's sleep, then this will have a major impact on the quality of your mood. There are a number of rules, many of which have been mentioned already:

- Get up at a regular time; the body likes routine.
- Eat at regular times; again, the body likes routine.
- Avoid too much caffeine (not more than around three cups of instant coffee per day) and too much alcohol (not more than three units per day if you are a man, two if you're a woman).
- Include a reasonable amount of physical and mental activity into your day; try to break the vicious circle

285

of feeling tired, therefore not doing much, therefore not sleeping very well and therefore feeling tired . . .

- Have a wind-down period before you go to bed; a low-activity routine so that you go to bed relaxed.
- Make sure you're neither too hungry nor too full when you go to bed.
- Ensure that you have a regular bedtime; again, the body likes routine.
- Some people find they are able to induce a state of happiness as they lie in bed; if you can do this it's a good idea – happy people sleep better than unhappy ones!
- Make sure you've got rid of any extraneous sudden noises from central heating or anything else, and that you are warm enough but not too hot.

Well, that may not be a comprehensive account of how to reform your sleeping habits, but it's a very good start. If you really make sure that you are doing all of those, all at once, then you shouldn't be sleeping too badly at all. Only one other thing; don't *try* to sleep – even if you just lie there awake but relaxed all night your brain will go into a different mode and you'll have a reasonable amount of rest, so long as you don't actually harass yourself trying to get to sleep.

Sleep project

- Regardless of whether you think of yourself as having sleep problems it is still an excellent idea to get as good a night's sleep as possible. The importance of a good night's sleep is difficult to overestimate.
- Therefore apply your mind to implementing as many of the aforementioned points as you can, including setting realistic times for bedtime and getting-up time in order to ensure that you have enough time in bed but not too much.
- Of course, if you work shifts, this can be a problem. Some people seem to be able to manage shift work quite easily, others not. In either case make sure that you get straight into the new routine as soon as your shift changes; the body isn't normally too upset about occasional changes in the routine as long as you then stick to it for a substantial period of time. Other people simply cannot tolerate, for example, night-shift work. If you are one of those then you might have to take more radical measures like seeing if you can find a job that doesn't entail night-working.

Come what may, make sure you do everything in your power to get a good night's sleep.

Illness

If you are going through a period of illness, then the chances are that this will affect your mood.

There may not be a lot you can do about this. Let's assume that you are doing all you can in terms of overcoming the illness, regardless of whether it's short-term or long-term, physical or mental.

What we are interested in here is your levels of, and tendency towards, irritability and anger. In that respect there is one major thing you can do: namely, when you find a person who's irritating you and you suspect it may be because of your illness, make sure you lay the blame clearly on your *illness*, not on the *person*. If you want to swear and curse at anything, do it at the illness rather than the person. And, that being the case, make sure it's under your breath! Or, better still, make sure you're out of earshot and then swear and curse at the illness as much as you like.

There is a very important general rule here: it is always good to lay the blame where it belongs rather than on some poor unfortunate who happens to be nearby!

There is just one illness I'd like us to look at more carefully, because it is so often associated with irritability and anger. And that illness is a mental one, namely depression.

Depression

My friend and colleague Paul Gilbert has written an extremely good book on *Overcoming Depression* in this series. However, just for the moment, rather than embark on reading a completely new book, allow me to give you a few tips. That is all they are; but just see if any of these fits your needs.

- Think less, do more. Thinking is one of the great traps in depression. Many people, when they find themselves feeling low, indulge in two types of unhelpful thinking. First, they dwell on and brood over their problems; and second, they 'introspect'
  – in other words, they think too much about where they might be going wrong. As a general rule, too much thinking doesn't do us good. Effectively, it digs us deeper into the swamp we are trying to climb out of. Action, on the other hand, is usually helpful. It doesn't particularly matter what the action is. Doing things of any sort seems to be a good idea.

- Envisage a future you want. Regardless of whether you are thinking short-term or long-term, next weekend or ten years hence, looking forward to a good future is a powerful anti-depressant. Have a clear picture of what it is you want; write it down or draw pictures of what you're after. But whatever you do, make sure that you have really clear images of the future that you want and how you might obtain it. And do it regularly; it's not a 'once and for all' activity.

- When you do think, be careful what you think *about*.

Sometimes people spend time thinking about things that make them unhappy. Sometimes the connection is obvious – thinking about sad things makes most people unhappy. Sometimes it is less obvious; you might, for example, spend time thinking about a good relationship you used to have, but when you stop thinking about it find that you have become unhappy. Try to be aware of what effect your thoughts have on you, and spend less time thinking about things that make you unhappy and more time thinking about things that make you happy.

- Get yourself a good routine with plenty of exercise and sleep, good nutrition and limited unhelpful drugs. We have probably said enough about this one, but if you get all those things right you're off to a terrific start.

- Act as if you are happy and relaxed. The way we walk, sit, stand and talk gives signals to the brain about how we are. So, it's a good idea to send 'non-depressed' signals to the brain. Try an experiment if you want. Normally, if you're feeling down, you'll be sitting in a depressed kind of way. If somebody came in and saw you, they'd say you *looked* depressed. So, right now, sit in a non-depressed way. Very quickly, almost immediately, you'll feel the difference. It is very difficult to sit non-depressed and yet *feel* depressed. If you act *as if* you're happy and relaxed, your brain will, to a degree, follow your lead.

• Have a *good day*. Life consists of a series of days; if you can make each one reasonably good, then you will have a rewarding life. Of course, most days involve some things we don't really want to do and other things we do want to do. The best slogan here is: 'Do the worst first.' That way you're always on the 'downhill run', each thing leading on to something better. If you do it the other way round, you are constantly being 'punished' for everything you do. Also, beware of trying to plan things that will make you happy: you are probably on to a loser here. Happiness is an elusive quality: the more you chase it, the more it runs away from you. It's maybe better to plan things that you think are 'right' or possibly even things that will 'make you feel good about yourself'.

• Sort out your environment. Sometimes when I call on people who have been depressed for a while, I look at where they live and think it's no wonder they're depressed. Any reasonable person, living there, would be depressed. And it's not usually anything to do with money; it's just a badly organised environment. There are three key principles:

(1) Arrange things so you feel safe (you're not going to trip up, electrocute yourself, bump into sharp corners, etc.); (2) have things so you are comfortable (chairs, bed, table, work surfaces); (3) have things around you that you like and that make you feel good (specific furniture, pictures, colours, etc.). Take this further if you want. Watch and listen to television and radio programmes that make you feel good rather than bad. Listen to music that makes you feel upbeat rather than down, and so on.

- Sort out your social life. Most people are social beings, so it's important to have this area reasonably well sorted. In the first place, intimate relationships are very important to us, so if you have one it's important to do your level best to make it as good as it can be. Work at developing a good relationship with your partner. For some people this isn't very good, but just get it to its maximum! One word of warning: if you are depressed, you tend to be depressed about your partner (in just the same way as you're probably also depressed with your house, job, car, etc.).

This does not mean that your partner is necessarily *causing* your depression. Of course, s/he may be; but be cautious, think carefully before you do or say anything too precipitate.

- Non-intimate relationships are important too. Make them as good as you can. But make them 'real' relationships. In other words, to paraphrase President Kennedy, 'Ask not what your friends can do for you, but what you can do for your friends.' Humans have a rather good design feature whereby if you follow that maxim, your friends benefit a lot *and so do you*. It's a question of cultivating a real interest in your friends rather than 'using them' to provide yourself with a social life.

- 'Gentle up' on yourself. Sometimes people can be really hard on themselves when they are depressed. In fact, sometimes it is the act of being so hard on themselves that causes the depression. They make rules for themselves that are rigid, extreme and overgeneralised, rules like: 'I've got to be loved by everybody', and 'I've got to be 100 per cent perfect in everything I do', and 'It's terrible if things aren't just the way I want them to be'. To lighten up on yourself, soften these rules to: 'It is nice to have some people who like me (but I can't be liked by everybody)', 'It is nice to do things right (but sometimes things are less than perfect)', 'I'd sooner have things go the way I want them (but then again, that's not always the way life is)'. The rules we make for ourselves are often almost unconscious, so sometimes we really have to work hard on softening them up.

Depression project

- If you feel you are depressed and your irritability is caused by your depression, then you need to sort your depression out.
- The points listed above are probably highly relevant for you. You need to tackle them methodically. In other words, choose just one of the factors above and really go to town on that one for the next week or two. And then choose another, and then another, until you've covered all the ones that you feel are relevant to you. This is a good major project because it will make you happier and less irritable. Indeed, it can be little short of life-transforming.
- If you want to do a more comprehensive job on your depression, then embark on Paul Gilbert's *Overcoming Depression* or David D. Burns's *The Feeling Good Handbook*, both of which are excellent. And there are other excellent ones too.

- Alternatively (or in addition), you can go along to your doctor; depression is so common that they normally have a good system for helping. Your doctor will also be vigilant for illnesses such as hypothyroidism which are physical in nature but whose symptoms mimic those of depression.
- In any case, it's a shame for you to go through life depressed, so set yourself a real project to resolve it. It can be done, even if you've been depressed for ages.

Tip

Remember, whether your illness is depression or some other affliction, maybe a physical condition, develop the habit whenever you feel irritable of blaming the illness, not the person who seems to be causing the irritation.

Life stresses

Stressful life events come in at least two sorts: repetitive stresses such as overwork; and 'once off' events such as bereavement and divorce. Both can affect our mood substantially.

Let's take the repetitive stresses first of all. We are talking here about things such as overwork, demanding family members (such as difficult children, or having to look after an ageing parent), or demanding friends who need your attention. Any one of these can become wearing; or pressure from two or more together can add up to the point where it has a serious effect on your mood.

There are three things you can do:

- Reduce the stresses
- Learn to cope with the stresses better
- View the stresses in a different light

We'll look at these briefly in turn in a moment, but before we do there is one other important point to be made. Again, as with illness, if you are feeling irritable because you are 'stressed out', make sure you put the blame where it belongs, in other words, on the stress: overwork, or whatever it happens to be. Don't displace it on to whoever happens to be closest to hand.

Take Nish, for example, our stressed-out executive. Nish is under stress because of his work, not his home life. Even so, because he's stressed, when he goes home to his wife Nadia, he is irritable. This means that almost anything Nadia does irritates Nish, not because *she is irritating* but because *he is irritable*. So Nish had to learn to snap *not* at Nadia but at his workload. He did this rather clumsily at first. Nadia would say something like, 'What should we do for dinner tonight?' and Nish, rather than replying, 'I don't care', in an irritable way, had to teach himself to say: 'All the stuff going on at work is getting me down.' This was pretty strange to Nadia at first, because it is a rather odd reply to 'What should we do for dinner tonight?' Nevertheless, Nish got better at it, and eventually was able to say it quietly to himself – making the point that he was stressed out not by Nadia but by his work. Further down the line he reduced his work pressures, which was of course the long-term solution. (But also see later on, about viewing stress in a different light.)

What I'm trying to say is: blame what deserves to be blamed, rather than the person in front of you. Then, better still, sort out the underlying problem.

So, here goes. The first course of action was to *reduce the stress*. Most people's first response to this is 'easier said than done', and there is some truth in that. For example, one woman I saw, Jasmin, had her mother living a few doors down from her, and the mother for very good reasons needed frequent attention. Jasmin said there was no way that she could give her mother any less attention than she did, so how could she possibly reduce the pressures on herself? And she seemed to be correct; her mother really did seem to need the attention described. However, as we talked I learnt that Jasmin was (a) holding down a fairly demanding job, (b) coming home to a husband and two children and setting about making a traditional evening meal from scratch, and (c), then going off to give her mother the attention she needed. In fact, she also managed to fit in a brief visit to her mother between coming home and setting about making the meal. So, although she had to continue to give her mother the same amount of attention, Jasmin could reduce the pressures on herself in other areas. She chose to cut down on the amount of work involved in making the meal. She couldn't quite bring herself to delegate it to her husband, but she did go for quicker, simpler dishes and ingredients, and that brought her total workload down to a manageable level.

Reducing stress

If you know you're being 'stressed out' by too many pressures, examine the total pressures you are under and do anything you can to reduce that total. The principal pressure may be unalterable, or alterable only to a small degree. Don't be put off by that; work on some of the other pressures you are under. Also, beware of blocking yourself by assuming that the major pressure is unalterable. Sometimes it isn't, even when it seems to be. Do some careful analysis and see where you can de-stress yourself.

The second course of action we looked at was *learning to cope with stresses better*. By this I mean you don't change the number or quantity of stresses affecting you; you simply act differently.

I feel that here I should start telling you about time management, self-instructional training and so forth. On the other hand, I don't know enough about what particular stresses *you* are under to make such a discussion directly relevant to you. So I will just suggest this:

- Try to clarify in your mind exactly what the stresses are (which can be more difficult than at first sight seems)
- Then ask several people you know how they cope with those stresses.

For example:

- If you get stressed out by putting two youngsters to bed, neither of whom wants to go and both of whom are liable to be naughty in lots of different ways, ask someone else you know how they cope with it. It doesn't have to be a contemporary of yours, though it can be if you prefer; it might be someone rather older who knows what they would do 'if they had their time again'.
- If you are stressed out by having three deadlines to meet and being aware that it is impossible to meet all three, ask somebody else who finds themselves in a similar situation what they do.

- If you are stressed out by having an over-energetic friend who always wants to drag you off to the latest new and exciting place, ask somebody else in a similar situation how they cope with that. Again, it does not have to be an exact parallel. The person you ask might have a friend who is always burdening them with their problems but has found a method for coping with that. Maybe you could still tailor their solution to your own situation.

- If you are stressed out by being jobless, wanting a job and having too much time on your hands, again ask other people in the same situation how they cope. Possibly, just possibly, you might be able to put together a solution from the various answers you receive.

Learning to cope with stress

- If you feel this is a relevant area for you, do your own 'research project' on how you might cope better with the stresses affecting you. This method hinges on:

- Being able to identify very clearly what it is that is stressing you.

- Being able to conduct a 'survey' of one or more people who might be able to offer you a solution or a partial solution.
- Putting together a personal plan that suits your own situation.
- Having the determination to implement that personal plan.

The third solution we had to life's stresses was to *view them in a different way*.

An example. I have a friend who has a soft spot for Bangladesh. He has a tremendous amount of empathy for the Bangladeshis and the sufferings they endure by way of floods, storms and winds. He is constantly devastated by the number of people who lose their lives in the country, the amount of suffering that goes on there, and he sends regular sums of money to aid programmes associated with Bangladesh.

However, he is far from solemn about this serious concern, and whenever he hits a problem, says, 'Compared with the problems they have in Bangladesh, this is no problem at all.' And, although he says it in a flippant kind of way, it clearly has a major impact on his thinking. It is his way of 'reframing' his own problems.

Obviously, this is simply a variant on the time-honoured admonition, 'There are plenty of people worse off than you.' However, it is a very good variant for my friend because it is so much more specific. My friend really does envisage in his own mind trying to explain his problem to somebody in Bangladesh, and how minor and trivial his own problem would seem to them. Very convincing reframing.

A step on from reframing – a more extreme form, even – is to question the long-held assumption that stress is bad for us. There is some remarkable research lately which suggests that it is not stress that is bad for us but *the belief that stress is bad for us* that is bad for us. A long-term study over many years, cited by Kelly McGonigal, demonstrated that people who are under high stress but didn't believe stress is bad for them lived longer than people who are under moderate stress. And the people who live shortest were those who are under high stress and believed that stress was bad for them. Personally I am delighted with this research because I have always lived a fairly high-stress life and thought that was a mistake, but it turns out that maybe that's not the case; it may not matter how much stress we are under so long as we don't have the idea that it does us harm. Remarkable research that I commend to you (see 'taking it further' at the end of the chapter.)

Reframing stress

- Reframing is a very powerful tool if you can get into it. It has the power to transform a situation quickly and permanently, if you're prepared to undertake it.

- Use the examples given above to see if there's a parallel in your own situation. How could you reframe your own situation?
- Note: This is not just an intellectual exercise! Once you have worked out how it is possible to reframe your own situation you then have to go ahead and do it. Get yourself in the habit of seeing your situation from this new viewpoint.

Social factors

Being social animals, we humans are greatly affected in our moods by how our social lives are progressing.

There are three major areas we have to consider:

- Our most intimate relationships: with our partners if we are adults, more probably with peers, parents or carers if we are children.
- Social relationships at work or wherever we occupy ourselves.
- Social relationships outside of intimate and work ones, namely with friends, neighbours, etc.

To maintain a good long-term mood we need to nurture each of these three areas as best we can: not just 'using' other people to provide ourselves with a social life, but taking a genuine interest in others to give ourselves a solid social foundation.

Inevitably, however, things go wrong in one area or another. For example, you might have trouble with your relationships at work – with your boss, with colleagues, with clients, or whoever. The most common mistake in this instance is to come home and be snappy with those at home. In other words, you transfer problems from one area into a second area, immediately doubling the problem.

An alternative habit is just as easy to get into. We have to take it as given that problems do sometimes arise, so that, inevitably, there will sometimes be difficulties in relationships at work, for example. It is then a question of disciplining ourselves to switch into a different 'gear' when we get home: a gear that appreciates the support of those with whom we live, or at least one that takes us into a totally different mode at home from that prevailing at work.

And the same applies the other way round: there are sometimes problems at home that don't need to be transferred to work or friendships. When one area temporarily goes down, we need to make sure we don't contaminate the other two areas.

This is exactly the trap that Maya was walking into. She was the teenager who was depressed and irritable because she had repeated problems with her boyfriends: so, at home, she would be snappy with her parents and her brother because of the 'boyfriend trouble'. In this way she was alienating the very people who would naturally have provided her with support.

Maya was a particularly interesting example to me because she grasped this concept straight away. This was very satisfying to me as a therapist, because I could see the immediate impact of her recognition. Immediately she realised what she was doing, she acted upon the idea that the times when she was sad about her boyfriend situation were the very times when she should put *more* energy into her (good) domestic situation, and the good relationships she had with other friends.

Social project

The project in this area has two parts:

- First, if necessary, build your social support in the three areas of intimate relationships: work relationships (if you go to work) and other relationships such as those with your neighbours and friends.
- Second, be constantly aware of the trap of displacing trouble from one of the three areas into another and thereby doubling or trebling your trouble. Skirt your way round this trap by acting upon the realisation that when you have trouble in one of the three areas, this is the very time to lean on and nurture the other two areas.

Summary

This has been a big chapter that has looked at the all-pervasive influence of our mood on irritability and anger. It is fluctuations in mood that lead to the unpleasant effect of 'just feeling irritable' with no apparent trigger. In fact, when you feel irritable, almost anything can trigger irritation.

But mood is not random. You can work to produce a good, stable mood by achieving the following:

- Develop a good circadian rhythm or daily routine, particularly in respect to eating and sleeping at regular times.
- Take exercise – any exercise!
- Eat a balanced diet, eat it well, and drink plenty of water.
- Go easy on caffeine (around three cups of instant coffee per day), alcohol, nicotine and other 'recreational' drugs.
- Develop a pattern of sound, refreshing sleep.
- If your irritable mood is due to illness, it's a question of clearing up the illness if possible, and if not then making sure you blame your irritability on the illness rather than on the people around you.
- Reduce the stressful effect of life stresses by (a) removing one or more of the stresses – not always the most obvious one; (b) learning to

cope with the stresses better, including by asking others how they cope with them; and/or (c) reframing the stresses, including realising that there is nothing especially wrong with stress unless you think there is!

- Nurture the three key areas in your social life and, when you have trouble in one of the three areas, ensure that you don't spread it to the other two.

Project

- A lot of individual projects have been set out in the course of this chapter. Your task now is an enjoyable one: read through the chapter, decide which are the most relevant areas for you, and undertake the project(s) described under that area.
- Raising your mood is a terrific task to undertake and a very rewarding one indeed. Not only will it make you less irritable, it will permanently brighten up everything around you!

Taking it further

To see a video talk of the research I mentioned about stress not being bad for us but *the belief that stress is bad for us* being bad for us, go to www.ted.com and search for Kelly McGonigal. The talk is entitled *How to make stress your friend* and it is excellent.

PART THREE

PUTTING THINGS INTO PRACTICE

We have come a long way; at the beginning of the book we were looking at the meanings of the words anger and irritability. Now we can comfortably look at a complex case and handle it with some confidence, so Part Three of this book is all about reaping the rewards: using what we have covered in order to make sense of an interesting case, and matching that up with you, or others you know.

24

A case study

It is important to be able to make sense of what makes us lose our temper or lose control of ourselves, so I want to describe an incident that we will look at. It was a major incident; Andy, the person concerned, describes how, when he had regained his temper, it was like having had a fit – it took him about forty-eight hours to regain his equilibrium. And in line with that, Stephanie (his wife) describes how he looked slightly strange for that period of time. This fits with the 'amygdala hijack' observation, where the brain is literally overwhelmed by an attack of anger. It may be familiar to many people reading this book.

My plan is to give you increasing layers of information and invite you to guess what caused Andy to lose his temper. Then I'll give you an analysis so you can see how your views compare with mine.

The incident took place in a small town on Cyprus called Paphos. Andy and his wife Stephanie were on holiday, and had called in to Paphos to see what it was like – they had been there some years previously. They stopped at a small cafe for lunch and, unusually for them, shared a lunchtime bottle of red wine. Both the lunch and the red wine were mildly disappointing and it was towards the end of lunch that Andy lost it big time, becoming very angry with Stephanie, saying 'terrible things' about her way beyond the apparent cause of the argument. Now, describing the incident two years later, he cannot even remember what the argument was about; the real issue was that, for whatever reason, he totally lost his temper.

Decision-point 1: What is your best guess as to why Andy lost his temper? Please write it down (preferably) or make a firm mental note of it before reading on.

Your next piece of information is that Andy's wife, Stephanie, says that she can remember perfectly well what the trigger was. She says it was hot and they were drinking and she made a comment about a great book they were reading; apparently she said that James, the person who recommended the book, of course would be able to recommend a good book because 'that's the sort of thing he is good at'. She says that Andy took it badly because he also had recommended a book to Stephanie and she had chosen to ignore that.

Decision-point 2: Now what is your best guess as to why Andy lost his temper? You may not have changed your view from your first guess, but on the other hand you may have. Again, please write down your current best guess, or make a firm mental note of it before reading on.

The next piece of information is that Andy and his wife Stephanie were on a cruise of the Eastern Mediterranean and neither of them had been sleeping particularly well for the last few days. Not terribly, but not particularly well. Also, the food on the ship wasn't quite as good as they were used to back home; they were both used to a good diet, and the ship's catering was necessarily geared to three thousand hungry people all wanting to eat at roughly the same time several times a day. Also they had both had a drink or two at lunchtime for the last three days, something they didn't usually do.

Decision-point 3: Now what is your best guess as to why Andy lost his temper? You may not have changed your view from your first guess, but on the other hand you may have. Again, please write down your current best guess (preferably), or make a firm mental note of it before reading on.

Your next piece of information is that, many years previously, Andy and Stephanie had their honeymoon in Paphos.

Decision-point 4: Now what is your best guess as to why Andy lost his temper? You may not have changed your view from earlier, but on the other hand you may have. Again, please write down your current best guess (preferably), or make a firm mental note of it before reading on.

Your next piece of information is that Andy, when he was seventeen, was involved in a tragic road accident in which he was seriously injured but his girlfriend was killed. He loved the girl very much, and also felt – and feels – partly responsible for the accident.

Decision-point 5: Now what is your best guess as to why Andy lost his temper? Please write down your current best guess (preferably), or make a firm mental note of it before reading on.

Your next piece of information is that when Andy and Stephanie honeymooned in this small town they had stayed in one of the cheaper hotels, although just along from the best hotel in town. They joked that when they could afford it later in life they would come back and stay in the top hotel. Before having lunch in the disappointing cafe with the disappointing red wine, they had both gone into this lovely hotel and, for whatever reason, hadn't quite felt able to order lunch in the posh restaurant. Hence, they went and found a cafe.

Decision-point 6: Now what is your best guess as to why Andy lost his temper? Please write down your current best guess (preferably), or make a firm mental note of it before reading on.

Your next piece of information is that Andy was eighteen years old when he met Stephanie, who was seventeen. This was just a year after Andy's accident. They went out for three years although they didn't see as much of each other as they might have done because Andy was at university in Edinburgh and Stephanie was at university in Newcastle. When Andy finished his degree most of his best friends got jobs outside of Edinburgh, so Andy was lonely. It was at this point that Stephanie said to him that unless they were going to get engaged she wanted to end the relationship because she wasn't getting any younger. So they got engaged, although Andy has always felt that Stephanie had slightly taken advantage of the moment.

Decision-point 7: Now what is your best guess as to why Andy lost his temper? Please write down your current best guess (preferably), or make a firm mental note of it before reading on.

Your next piece of information is that on the day in question (the day that Andy lost his temper in such a big way) Andy was in his sixty-third year and Stephanie in her sixty-second. In other words, they had been married for about forty years.

Decision-point 8: Now what is your best guess as to why Andy lost his temper? Please write down your current best guess, or make a firm mental note of it before reading on.

Your next piece of information is that Andy had an affair about twenty or twenty-five years ago, starting when he was about thirty-five and finishing when he was in his early forties. He describes it as a very serious affair with a woman who reminded him of his girlfriend at seventeen. Stephanie knew about it and they came very close to separating so that he could go off with this other woman.

Decision-point 9: Now please write down your final best guess as to why Andy lost his temper, or make a firm mental note of it before reading on.

How did you get on? Typically people go through various stages, first of all being very clear on what caused Andy to lose his temper, then more uncertain, and then often demanding yet more information before feeling able to make a decision of any sort. Here is one record at the various decision points:

Decision point 1. This is just a case of a holiday argument, the result of not enough sleep and more drink than you're used to drinking.

Decision point 2. Yes, maybe Stephanie was a bit tactless, but basically this is just a holiday argument.

Decision point 3. This just confirms my original decision: they're both a bit tired, make the mistake of drinking halfway through the day when they don't really want to, and it all blows up.

Decision point 4. I'm sticking with my opinion, I think the fact that they honeymooned here years ago is not relevant.

Decision point 5. That's all very sad but probably not relevant, after all it says it was 'many years ago' so presumably Andy and Stephanie have been married for many years.

Decision point 6. Yes, this confirms me in my original view that it is just one of those holiday things: you're a bit tired, you have too much to drink, things don't turn out quite the way you wanted them to (in this case you don't end up in the hotel you wanted to have your lunch in), you end up in some disappointing cafe, and then everything blows up in your face.

Decision point 7. Actually this could throw a different light on it. Maybe there is an element of bitterness in Andy's mind and this has come to the fore now that they are back in the honeymoon destination.

Decision point 8. No, it looks as though I was right all along; surely Andy can't have been harbouring this bitterness for forty years?

Decision point 9. Again, this throws a new light on it. Maybe he has indeed been harbouring bitterness. Or maybe he just wishes he had gone off with this other woman. And it all comes to a head in a tired and disappointing drunken lunch at their honeymoon destination. But this other woman was twenty-five years ago, so surely he has got over her by now? But maybe not. I don't know. I would need to have some more information.

In fact the question 'Why did Andy lose his temper?' is a difficult one to answer. It seems like a straightforward question at first sight but, as we have seen, it gets more difficult the more thoroughly you look at it. And, if you look at the times that *you* lose your temper, you will see exactly the same thing. At first sight the reason seems obvious but then, as you look at it more carefully, it seems less and less obvious.

So I want us to look at a robust system based on the case formulation that top-rank mental health professionals use. And it is easy enough; what we do is to break the question down into two parts:

1. What predisposes the person to lose their temper? That is, what are the factors in the person's background that make them ready to explode given the right trigger?
2. What precipitates people losing their temper? That is, what is the trigger for the explosion?

Later on I'm going to invite you to examine one of your own explosions, but let's practice on Andy first. (Incidentally, at first sight it sounds rude to talk about your 'explosions' or, indeed, Andy's explosions. But I'm not convinced it is, because when you look at the flare up of neuronal firing when someone loses their temper, it really is akin to an explosion.)

So, considering Andy, what were the predisposing factors – the factors that meant that he was ready to explode given the right trigger? Here are some possibilities:

1. He had a tragic car accident at age seventeen which might have resulted in post-traumatic stress disorder and may also have resulted in 'complicated grief' at the loss of his girlfriend. So maybe any subsequent

wife or girlfriend was going to be on 'thin ice'. Especially maybe when revisiting the scene of their honeymoon.

2. We also know that it was hot, Andy hadn't been sleeping very well for the last few nights, had not been receiving good nutrition, and had been drinking some (substandard?) wine. These are all much more recent factors than the car accident at seventeen, and maybe they seem more 'superficial' things, but they are certainly factors which are going to predispose him to 'explode' given the right trigger. (We have seen these biological factors in the chapter on Mood.)

3. There may also be some 'thinking errors' in play. For example, perhaps he has an exaggerated idea of 'idealised love'. So, maybe he imagines that if he had married his seventeen-year-old girlfriend, or maybe his later mistress, that they would have lived the most amazingly happy life evermore, a life happier than could be imagined. In reality, who knows, maybe that would have happened but, also, maybe she would have left him for somebody else after five years. It's impossible for us – or Andy – to know. It is, however, quite possible for Andy to imagine that would have been the case!

Or, if indeed he does have an exaggerated idea of 'idealised love' it may take a less extreme form. For example, he may have been attracted to the idea that when he and his wife returned to their honeymoon venue years later they would be wealthy enough to go to the best hotel and order a slap-up lunch. When, in reality, they either couldn't do this or didn't feel like doing it, this may have been a big disappointment, shattering a dream.

Or maybe the thinking error was not that at all but, instead, was an idea that Andy had that he must above all provide his wife with a really good income and standard of living. Then, to return to their place of honeymoon after forty years and find that they had only 'progressed' as far as a substandard cafe serving poor food and wine had a significance out of proportion.

So there are certainly some important factors that predisposed Andy to explode. But what were the factors that precipitated it – triggered it?

1. It looks like one trigger was the substandard meal, cafe and wine. Of course, at any other time this would not have acted as a trigger; Andy says he's been to plenty of substandard cafes and had disappointing meals before.

2. The trigger that Andy's wife recollects is a comment she made about a book they were reading – in fact she was reading it to him during the holiday and they were enjoying it greatly. It had been recommended to them by a friend, James, and Stephanie had commented that he of course would be able to recommend a good book, as 'it is the sort of thing he is good at'. Andy took offence that he also had

322

recommended a book to Stephanie and she had taken no notice – she had acted on James's recommendation instead.

So, in answer to the question 'What caused Andy to lose his temper?' we can give a full answer:

The immediate cause was a comment that his wife made that implied that a friend of theirs was more likely to make a good recommendation of a book to read than Andy was.

Moreover, it was at a time when Andy and his wife had not been sleeping well, they had been drinking at lunchtime for several days, it was hot, and their nutrition had been of lower quality than usual.

Stephanie's comment was also exacerbated because it occurred during a visit to a disappointing cafe, serving disappointing food and wine. This all had particular significance because it took place in the small town in which they had honeymooned forty years previously, so it seemed as though they had made remarkably little progress in forty years, moving from a cheap hotel then to a cheap cafe now. To rub salt into the wounds, after forty years it appeared that Stephanie was more inclined to trust the opinion of a friend than the opinion of Andy when it came to choosing a book to read. Maybe he wished that he had married the girl who died in the car accident many years before, or even the woman with whom he had had an affair more recently but still twenty years ago.

And yet it could easily have been so different: if only they had been lunching in the nearby posh hotel they could have congratulated themselves on the progress they had made, moving over the course of their marriage from cheap hotel to being on a cruise and eating at the best restaurant in town, having acquired urbane friends who could make incisive recommendations on the literature that would appeal to them. Such a small action could have made a big difference. Equally, if only Andy had not had such idealised ideas about how marriage should be it could also have been so different.

So we can understand why Andy lost his temper, at least in the sense that we can describe the sequence of events and why these were likely to have the effect they did on Andy. But of course Andy wants not to lose his temper like this in future so, to help him, what advice could we give? What advice would you give him? Here are some options:

1. Dump Stephanie, and go and find the woman you had an affair with twenty years ago and see if she will have you back.

2. Rearrange your ideas about marriage; marriage was never meant to be a fairy tale; so long as you're both reasonably healthy and happy then that is a good result.

3. Keep Stephanie if she'll have you, and keep your ideas about marriage. After all, it seems that you were on a decent cruise, and able to lunch in the best hotel in town if you had chosen to do so. And she was reading to you a good book recommended by your sophisticated friend. This has to be a good result by

any standards, so just recognise that. If you get some good nights' sleep, refrain from drinking on several lunchtimes in a row when you're on holiday in a hot climate, and eat an ordinarily decent diet and maybe get some exercise, then all of those things will help you see things more clearly. Then, if ever Stephanie makes what you take to be a tactless comment, you are less likely to overreact. After all, you probably make tactless comments as well sometimes.

4. Don't make so much of it; in the battle between what you do and what you think, always look at what you are doing first. So, if you're going to go back to your honeymoon destination after forty years then you can either hang around the same haunts as you did when you were on honeymoon, just to reminisce and remember good times, or you can go to the best restaurant in town and live it up. What you don't do is to go to some random cheap cafe and start boozing in the midday sun. If you do that and the slightest thing goes wrong, then you're bound to be in trouble. And the same thing applies wherever you are and whatever you're doing; you need to see things reasonably clearly and act accordingly.

Which of those would you choose? There isn't really a right answer although my favourite is number (4). Equally, numbers (2) and (3) are good as well. When you are seeing a patient you can't really recommend number one, although occasionally somebody will come to their own conclusion in that regard.

Does this case remind you of yourself in any way? If so, how?

25

Shutting the stable door does at least stop the rest of the horses from bolting

The aviation industry has been phenomenally successful in ensuring that flying is as safe as it possibly can be. Within the space of a hundred years we have seen flying transform from an activity where pioneers risked – and lost – their lives on a regular basis to a time when literally millions of people fly safely around the world in thousands of planes which manage never to crash or bump into each other. So it is worth looking at the systems they have in place to achieve this.

The first thing I want us to look at is known as 'shutting the stable door after the horse has bolted'. In other words, every time there is a 'major incident' they examine the incident in minute detail and see what lessons can be learned. Not so that they can turn the clock back, but so that the same thing doesn't happen again. And they do this in the spirit of 'no fault, and no blame' so that everybody concerned can be as open as possible. This is just the spirit in which we should examine our own breakdowns, without blaming ourselves or others.

This gives us a tremendous model to copy. It also gives us a silver lining to the cloud of losing our temper. Of course it is bad news to lose our temper, but if it is something we can learn from, improve from, and make future similar instances less likely, then at least some good will come out of it.

Therefore, the principle is good, so let's go back to Andy from the previous chapter and see how it applies in practice. And we have already done a lot of the work, we have already analysed the incident in some detail, so we are ready to answer the key question, which is: What can Andy do from now on to make similar events less likely to happen?

Exercise

After an air crash, the authorities compile a report making recommendations about actions that should be taken to prevent a similar event happening again. In the same spirit, which of the following are recommendations you would make to Andy, to minimise the chances of him having a similar incident again? Circle either Yes or No for each of the possible recommendations below. Bear in mind your recommendations are for Andy specifically, not for people in general.

1. Don't have a tragic car accident at age seventeen.

    Recommendation? Yes / No

2. Do your best to get a good night's sleep.

    Recommendation? Yes / No

3. Try to ensure you get good nutrition.

   Recommendation? Yes / No

4. Don't drink (substandard wine) in hot climates at lunchtime.

   Recommendation? Yes / No

5. Avoid having a mistress.

   Recommendation? Yes / No

6. Don't have overambitious ideas about how things are going to be when you've been married for forty years and return to your honeymoon destination.

   Recommendation? Yes / No

7. Don't have overinflated ideas about the income and standard of living you're going to provide for your wife.

   Recommendation? Yes / No

8. Don't go to substandard cafes.

   Recommendation? Yes / No

9. Don't allow Stephanie to make tactless remarks, either about friends recommending books or about anything else.

   Recommendation? Yes / No

10. Don't mind what books your wife reads.

    Recommendation? Yes / No

11. Don't let James ever recommend books for Stephanie to read.

    Recommendation? Yes / No

12. Make sure you eat in posh hotels.

    Recommendation? Yes / No

13. Go and find the woman you had an affair with twenty years ago and see if she will have you back.

    Recommendation? Yes / No

14. Rearrange your ideas about marriage; marriage was never meant to be a fairy tale; so long as you're both reasonably healthy and happy then that is a good result.

    Recommendation? Yes / No

15. Develop a better awareness of the situation you are in – for example, in this instance you were revisiting your honeymoon destination with your wife of forty years – and try to match your behaviour with the situation, whatever the situation is.

    Recommendation? Yes / No

In making your recommendations you might wish to bear in mind two potholes to skirt around:

1. Anything that necessitates turning the clock back can't be a recommendation, simply because we can't go back in time.
2. Anything that hinges on people other than Andy doing things can't be recommendations for Andy.

Now please put your recommendations in order so that, if Andy asks, 'What is your top recommendation?' Or 'What are your top three recommendations?' then you have a ready answer. This parallels aviation yet again: very often the authorities do not implement all of the recommendations made by the enquiry, just the most important ones. So, put '1' by your most important recommendation above, and so on.

Incidentally, the 'right answers' for this exercise are at the end of this chapter, but I suggest you don't look at them until you have thoroughly made up your own mind what you think.

Meantime, you may be thinking to yourself that you don't necessarily want to wait for major incidents to occur before you can improve yourself. Well, don't worry, because the aviation industry thinks exactly the same: they don't want to wait for aeroplanes to crash into each other before they do good things. In fact, what they do is to analyse 'near misses'. And we can do exactly the same.

What this means for us is that we analyse times where we didn't actually lose our temper 'big-time' but we came some way towards it. For example, in the case of Andy, the incident we have been examining was a truly major event. It took him about forty-eight hours to come down from it, and it is the most memorable episode of the eastern Mediterranean holiday. If you have events like that then you will be very familiar with how it is; and equally if you live with somebody who has events like that then you will be just as familiar. So how many times can we expect Stephanie to put up with these? Obviously Andy needs to work on himself in between such events. And we can all do exactly the same by spotting our own 'near-misses' and analysing them as though they were major incidents.

Meanwhile, here are the 'right answers' for the exercise.

1. Don't have a tragic car accident at age seventeen.

    No, this can't be a recommendation because we can't turn the clock back; we have to start from where we are now.

2. Do your best to get a good night's sleep.

    Yes, this is a recommendation because we know this is a factor in anger management and it clearly seems to have been a factor in this case.

3. Try to ensure you get good nutrition.

    Yes, this can be a recommendation, for the same reason.

4. Don't drink (substandard wine) in hot climates at lunchtime.

Yes, this can certainly be a recommendation. Apart from being straightforward common sense it was clearly a factor in this incident.

5. Avoid having a mistress.

No, this can't be a recommendation because again we can't turn the clock back.

6. Don't have overambitious ideas about how things are going to be when you've been married for forty years and return to your honeymoon destination.

No, this can't be a recommendation because even if Andy had had different ideas it may well not have prevented the incident happening.

7. Don't have overinflated ideas about the income and standard of living you're going to provide your wife with.

No, this isn't a recommendation for Andy because it appears they have actually done quite well financially so this wasn't really a factor. For other people it might be, and maybe as a general philosophy of life too.

8. Don't go to substandard cafes.

No, this can't be recommendation because Andy told us in his testimony that he frequently used substandard cafes, and in this enquiry we are trying to use 'logical, evidence-based reasoning'. Logically, if he goes to substandard cafes and doesn't lose his temper, then this can't be a major factor.

9. Don't allow Stephanie to make tactless remarks, either about friends recommending books or about anything else.

No, this can't be a recommendation because it relies on somebody else's behaviour. One of our rules for recommendations is that it has to concern our own behaviour only; it mustn't rely on what anybody else does.

10. Don't mind about what books Stephanie reads.

No, this is picking up on a detail that isn't particularly relevant.

11. Don't let James ever recommend books for Stephanie to read.

No, this can't be a recommendation because, again, it relies on somebody else's behaviour.

12. Make sure you eat in posh hotels.

No, Andy has told us that they eat in all sorts of places and he doesn't get angry as a result. There are other factors at play in this particular incident.

13. Go and find the woman you had an affair with twenty years ago and see if she will have you back.

No, it is difficult to recommend this because we have no idea what's happened to that woman and in any case Andy and Stephanie get on perfectly happily most of the time.

14. Rearrange your ideas about marriage; marriage was never meant to be a fairy tale; so long as you're both reasonably healthy and happy then that is a good result.

No, we examined this one and it doesn't really seem to be one that holds up.

15. Develop a better awareness of the situation you are in – for example, in this instance you were revisiting your honeymoon destination with your wife of forty years – and try to make your behaviour match the situation, whatever the situation is.

Yes, this is an important observation and highlighted an area that Andy was particularly weak on. He was relentless with himself and expected himself to behave consistently and reliably under all circumstances. This is not how life is; we are meant to look around us, assess the situation and behave in keeping with that situation. This is what he spectacularly failed to do in this instance, and in others as well. It was a major area of development for Andy.

The order I suggest the top three should go in is as follows:

1. Don't drink (substandard wine) in hot climates at lunchtime.

   The cost – benefit ratio of this one is so immense. It's not a difficult one to do (we know that Andy doesn't normally drink at lunchtimes), so why choose to do so in hot climates? The payoff should be great.

2. Do your best to get a good night's sleep and eat a good diet.

   Again, why wouldn't you get a good night's sleep and eat well? What is the argument against it? It's a nice thing to do and will have a payoff in terms of regulating emotions.

3. Develop a better awareness of the situation you are in – for example, in this instance you were revisiting your honeymoon destination with your wife of forty years – and try to make your behaviour fit the situation, whatever the situation is.

   This is my personal favourite and I'm disappointed to see it in third place even though I have put it there. This was a terrific one for Andy to work on, but of course it did require a significant amount of practice for him to get better at it. Even so, the payoff was great for him.

In fact, the most successful strategy we found for this was for Andy to notice the times when he was feeling *mildly* angry or irritated and to look at whether his behaviour was congruent to the situation. For example, he described how some disappointing news arrived one day and he responded by not changing his behaviour at all, in other words simply by carrying on with his work as though nothing had happened. Then he found himself doing substandard work which made him cross with himself, which made matters worse still. It was at that point that he asked himself whether the he was behaving congruently to the situation. Clearly he wasn't; he had given himself no time to cope with his disappointment before getting back to work again. In this instance he just took a mere two minutes out to give himself a break and come to terms with the news, before he got back to work again, but that two minutes made all the difference. Numerous examples like that improved his ability to monitor the situation and act accordingly.

Also a metaphor helped: Andy was a keen driver so we discussed the wisdom of driving straight ahead at a steady 50 miles an hour regardless of road conditions. He laughed at the very idea of this, saying that obviously you steer to the left and right and vary your speed according to what's going on. Fortunately, he could see how this principle applied to the rest of life as well.

26

Focusing on yourself

So we have now done quite a thorough job on Andy, probably as good or better job than you would find in most clinical settings. So let's see now whether you can do the same kind of job on yourself!

It should prove to be an interesting task for you, analysing one of your own 'incidents' in just the same way as we analysed Andy's, so let's recap on what to do:

1. Bring to mind a recent incident where you lost your temper. (Or, if you prefer, a 'near miss' where you nearly lost it.)
2. Get paper and pen – or use your computer or hand-held device – and write down the precipitating factors for you losing your temper in this particular instance. These are the 'triggers'. (In Andy's case the main trigger was a tactless remark from his wife.)
3. Write down the predisposing factors for you losing your temper in this particular instance. In Andy's case there were a number. For instance: drinking rough wine in a hot climate when he didn't normally drink at lunchtimes at all; having had some bad

nights' sleep two or three nights running; not eating a nutritious diet for a few days; and not behaving in a way that was congruent to the situation – in other words, going to a rough and ready cafe when revisiting their honeymoon destination forty years on! You might well find these predisposing factors particularly interesting in your own case, whatever they are; they tend to be the factors that most people overlook and yet they are probably the most important ones; even more important than the trigger, which is the one that people normally focus on.

4. Undertake an aviation-style enquiry into the incident, writing a list of recommendations that would prevent this same incident ever happening again.
5. Put your list of recommendations in the best order.
6. Make sure you act on your recommendations!

Writing this, I now feel bereft, because I would love to be alongside you and seeing what you have written, and to stay alongside you and see you act on your recommendations. If by any chance you have not done this exercise and have simply carried on reading what you're meant to do, then I would urge you to go back and actually complete it; hopefully you will find it tremendously beneficial. And, if you do it each time you either lose your temper or come close to it, then your temper is fighting a losing battle! What I mean by that is each time it raises its ugly head it is less likely to do so in the future, thanks to your analysis and action.

Finally, maybe just three 'tips' are in order:

A. Make sure you go through this procedure every time you lose your temper or come close to doing so. When we lose our temper it is never good news, but performing your analysis means that the very act of losing your temper makes it less likely to happen again, which has to be a good result.

B. Pay particular attention to the 'predisposing factors'. These are much easier to work on than the precipitating factors or 'triggers'. And, when you work on them, they typically have a really good benefit for you. Moreover, they sometimes don't take much work. (Remember, with Andy, the biggest recommendation was not to drink rough wine in hot weather on holiday at lunchtime which, given that he didn't normally drink at lunchtime, was not much effort for him. Nevertheless, if he follows this recommendation it is unlikely the same thing will happen to him again.)

C. Make sure you follow through on your recommendations. In other words, after you have done the analysis and you can see the actions you should take, be sure to take those actions. This sounds obvious, but sometimes we feel so pleased with ourselves having done such a good analysis, that we fall at the last hurdle by omitting to take the great action that we can see is necessary. Ironically, this may be especially so when the action is a simple one.

So good luck with this; if you can get anything like competent at this sort of analysis and action, you can do things which are likely to literally transform your life. I would love to be there to see it happen.

27

Troubleshooting guide

If you want to be less irritable and angry I suggest the following, in no particular order:

Address biological factors:

This might seem a bit basic but on the other hand if you have a good night's sleep, eat well, take some exercise, maintain a daily routine (going to bed at roughly the same time most nights and getting up at the same time most mornings, and eating meals at roughly the same time every day), it is surprising how much less irritable you can be. And if you are less irritable you end up less angry. If you do all of these things and find it has a really good result, don't assume you are now cured; if you let go of your new good habits then you will go back to square one.

Equally, if you are in any way ill, either with a short-term illness or long-term illness, this is likely to make you more irritable. So clearly you would try to get it resolved and, in any event, when you feel the inevitable irritability, make sure you blame the illness and not those around you!

Have a look at what you are doing

When we get irritable and angry we tend to focus on other people, and what they have done to make us this way. Often enough we can prevent things getting to this stage by changing what we ourselves are doing. For instance:

- I have really enjoyed writing this book, so I was surprised one day to find that I was working on it and not enjoying it – feeling a bit irritable in fact. Not helped by having a cold, not having slept well the previous night, and not having had any exercise for a few days thanks to the cold. So what is the best thing to do? Soldier on, cursing my irritability? I think not. Best to give it a miss and come back to it later or the next day.

- Often enough people just get bored, because they can't think of anything they want to do, and being bored is irritating. After all, what is life but what we do? If this rings a bell for you, I have put a list of possible things to do in the Appendix. It's a list I've taken a while to compile, so there are a lot of things on it – there should be one that is right for you at any particular time.

- Certain people's jobs really get them down. I know one person who regularly comes home completely worn down by their job and only just has enough energy left to be irritable with those around her. Sometimes it is possible to make small but significant changes to the job that produce an improvement for you. Other times it's actually worth changing the work you do, but don't try this is a first resort; try everything else first, because it could be that your irritability is being projected onto the job, rather than the job causing the irritability.

Maybe those examples ring a bell, maybe not. Either way it's always worth having a look at what you are doing: the solution isn't always biological or psychological; sometimes it's just a matter of doing something different. If the kids next door are irritating you by playing soccer outside the house and your normal reaction is to sit indoors and fume, then maybe – just maybe – you might be better off going out and playing ball with them.

Respond to your emotions

Everybody sometimes gets sad, worried, disappointed, grieves, feels upset and so on. Fortunately, if we wait long enough, good positive emotions will also strike us! When we are in one of these negative states, of course we are all likely to be irritable and get angry with people and things, but this is made worse if we don't recognise we are in a bad way and act accordingly. What does 'act accordingly' mean? It normally means being extra nice to ourselves, not expecting too much of ourselves. Paul Gilbert writes well about compassion-focused therapy and his point is a good one: we need to learn to be compassionate to ourselves.

Be sensitive to the surroundings

Sometimes it is very clear what the trigger for your irritability is; maybe it is the fact of the house being untidy, or the car being dirty, or – in a restaurant – that there is a cold draft that comes in every time somebody enters the restaurant. If you know what the trigger is and you can get rid of it, then it's a good idea to do so. Maybe you can tidy the house, clean the car, move to a different table in the restaurant.

Sometimes is not a question of the physical surroundings though, it is the people surrounding you who you find irritating! The same thing applies, though: if you can get away from those people then that is probably a good thing to do (and equally, if you can't, then try one of the other things we catalogue here).

Think about your thinking

There are quite a few enjoyable tricks we can play here, and these are some of them:

- You can alter the way you look at something. For instance, occasionally we will think that somebody is winding us up deliberately, whereas in fact this rarely happens – it's usually just accidental.
- Know when you have become sensitised to something. This is where you are grossly oversensitive to what is really only a small thing – your partner speaking with his or her mouth full of food, for example; the sort of

thing you hardly notice when you first meet but, after living with it for twenty years, can drive you crazy. What you need to do here (with thanks to Alcoholics Anonymous and apologies for the paraphrasing) is: to change it if you can change it, to live with it if you can't change it, and to know whether it is something that can be changed or can't be changed.

- Rule-governed behaviour. We all have rules that govern our behaviour and we make them up for ourselves. So, for example, most of us will have a rule that we don't murder people no matter how angry we are with them, and the fact that we have this rule prevents us from doing it. We can equally make up a rule like, 'I will never shout at anybody through anger'. Good rules are all or nothing (never / always etc). They are also thought through, so in this case the rule allows you to shout at people to warn them of an approaching vehicle, but not because you are angry.

- You can alter the way you think about anger. For instance, some people think it is good to 'let it out' whereas when they examine it carefully they find that 'letting anger out' is rarely a pleasant experience, either for them or for those around them. In fact anger just leaks away over time; there's no need to let it out – it goes away of its own accord.

- People indulge in 'recreational anger' because it makes them feel so energised, so alive and so right. Recreational anger is where you spend time thinking how wronged you have been and what great action you are going to take to put it right. This is a dangerous path to tread because the anger distorts your judgement as it comes from the less-developed part of the brain. You are better off taking your grievance to a trusted friend to ask their advice – and taking it.

- You can decide what your overarching life principles are – the kind of things you would like someone to say about you at a big birthday celebration – and be intent on living your life by them. The sense of direction this gives us is often very helpful in regulating how we feel and act.

- We can work on what we believe about other people. For example, if we think that other people are generally hostile and unhelpful then we are more likely to get angry with them than if we think that other people are generally helpful and supportive. The trouble with this one is that we think our beliefs are actual facts. In other words, because we believe people are hostile and unhelpful we think they actually ARE hostile and unhelpful. In reality, just because we believe something to be true it doesn't make it true and it's a good exercise to see if we can change what we believe. It can take a while, but it's time well spent.

Get expert on your anger

Again, this is interesting because it involves us thinking about ourselves. There are several way of becoming expert on your anger:

- Keep a diary, maybe using the diary forms in this book (there are extra copies in the Appendix), so you can see what makes you irritable and angry. Knowledge is power: if you know what makes you irritable and angry, then it's often clear what you should do about it.

- When you have an episode of anger or irritability, analyse it. Ask yourself what made you vulnerable to becoming angry at that point (for example, were you tired, or hungry, or had had too much to drink)? What sparked off the episode – what triggered it (for example, somebody's tactless comment). What else might you have done? What could you do to prevent it happening again next time? (This is a key question, one you need to act on.)

- Examine 'near misses' (where you didn't actually get angry but came close to it) in the same way. This is an excellent source of information and if you act on your conclusions it will do very well for you.

- Examine times when you are pleased you managed to stay ordinary in the face of something that might normally have made you angry. Analyse it so you can see what you did to achieve this. Whatever it was, do it again next time!

Treat yourself with compassion and respect.

Sometimes, when we get angry, it wears down the compassion and respect we feel for ourselves afterwards. This is a pity for two reasons: firstly it's an unpleasant feeling for us, and secondly it doesn't work well. It turns out that it usually works better when we guide ourselves in a supportive and compassionate way than when we harangue and criticise ourselves.

If you are applying this to a friend

I know that a lot of people buy this book in order to help a close friend or relative, and that's a splendid idea, and it is clear how you should use it – simply apply the sections you think are most relevant, or help your loved one to apply them. Just one last tip: 'validation' is rightly fashionable in the profession, and what it means in anger and irritability is that it is sometimes helpful to agree with the person who is angry rather than trying to calm them down. Occasionally, trying to calm them down actually ends up making things worse. As ever, an example. We live near a school and I get irritated by the fact that often enough a parent will park their car obstructing the entrance and exit of our drive. It doesn't bother my wife, but instead of reassuring me this irritates me still more. What I really want her to do is to say, 'Yes, it's really irritating isn't it, people have got no consideration for others, I feel like going out and giving them a good piece of my mind.' If she did say this I would probably do my best to reassure and calm her down, and all would be well!

Good Luck!

I hope you've enjoyed reading this book and, more to the point, I hope you have found it useful. I have certainly enjoyed writing it and confess to being pleased with the result. I think you have all the information here necessary to sort out your irritability or anger successfully and permanently.

Maybe, indeed, you have done so already, just in the course of your first reading. This is especially likely if you have chosen the projects carefully for yourself and implemented them thoroughly.

A word of caution and encouragement, however. Old habits die hard, and you may very well find that you have to reread parts of this book over months and even years to maintain your success. Indeed, I would urge you to do that, because the more pieces of the jigsaw you get in place, the easier it is to see a good clear picture. It may be that, when you first read through the book, you just 'cream off' the most relevant bits for yourself. On rereading you might implement other bits that are relevant, but not quite so relevant as the first level. This is still well worth doing, however, because it makes the whole process clearer and easier. So, do reread, lots of times if you want, because the projects are good ones and will really sort things out for you if you follow them through.

And one final thought: You probably embarked on this book out of consideration for those around you – and very commendable that is. Nevertheless, I hope you find that it has done wonders for your own enjoyment of life, too!

APPENDIX

Diary 1

Keep a record of when you get irritable or angry. Fill it in as soon as possible after the event. Note as clearly as possible what triggered your irritability/anger, and how you responded.

Trigger (include day, date and time)

Response (what did you do?)

Diary 1

Fill in as soon as possible after the event.

Trigger (include day, date and time)

Response (what did you do?)

Diary 1

Fill in as soon as possible after the event.

> **Trigger** (include day, date and time)

> **Response** (what did you do?)

Diary 1

Fill it in as soon as possible after the event.

Trigger (include day, date and time)

Response (what did you do?)

Diary 1

Fill it in as soon as possible after the event.

Trigger (include day, date and time)

Response (what did you do?)

Diary 2

Fill this in as soon as possible after each time you get irritable or angry.

Trigger: Describe here what a video camera would have seen or heard. Include the day and date, but do not put what you thought or how you reacted.

_____

_____

_____

_____

Appraisal/Judgement: Write here the thoughts that went through your mind, as clearly as you can remember them.

_____

_____

_____

_____

Anger: Leave this blank for the time being.

_____

_____

_____

_____

Inhibitions: Leave this blank for the time being.

_____

_____

_____

_____

Response: Write here what a video camera would have seen you do and heard you say, as clearly as you can.

_____

_____

_____

_____

More helpful appraisal/judgement: How else might you have appraised the situation? To determine this, you might like to consider the following: What errors are you making (selective perception, mind-reading, all or nothing thinking, emotive language, overgeneralisation)?

_____

_____

_____

_____

If you had an all-knowing, all-wise friend, how would s/he have seen the situation?

Is a reframing of the situation possible? (A glass that is half empty is also half full.)

What would your cost–benefit analysis be of seeing the situation the way you did?

_____

_____

_____

_____

Diary 2

Fill this in as soon as possible after each time you get irritable or angry.

Trigger: Describe here what a video camera would have seen or heard. Include the day and date, but do not put what you thought or how you reacted.

_____

_____

_____

_____

Appraisal/Judgement: Write here the thoughts that went through your mind, as clearly as you can remember them.

_____

_____

_____

_____

Anger: Leave this blank for the time being.

_____

_____

_____

_____

Inhibitions: Leave this blank for the time being.

_____

_____

_____

_____

Response: Write here what a video camera would have seen you do and heard you say, as clearly as you can.

_____

_____

_____

_____

More helpful appraisal/judgement: How else might you have appraised the situation? To determine this, you might like to consider the following: What errors are you making (selective perception, mind-reading, all or nothing thinking, emotive language, overgeneralisation)?

_____

_____

_____

_____

If you had an all-knowing, all-wise friend, how would s/he have seen the situation?

Is a reframing of the situation possible? (A glass that is half empty is also half full.)

What would your cost–benefit analysis be of seeing the situation the way you did?

_____

_____

_____

_____

Diary 2

Fill this in as soon as possible after each time you get irritable or angry.

Trigger: Describe here what a video camera would have seen or heard. Include the day and date, but do not put what you thought or how you reacted.

_____

_____

_____

_____

Appraisal/Judgement: Write here the thoughts that went through your mind, as clearly as you can remember them.

_____

_____

_____

_____

Anger: Leave this blank for the time being.

_____

_____

_____

_____

Inhibitions: Leave this blank for the time being.

_____

_____

_____

_____

Response: Write here what a video camera would have seen you do and heard you say, as clearly as you can.

_____

_____

_____

_____

More helpful appraisal/judgement: How else might you have appraised the situation? To determine this, you might like to consider the following: What errors are you making (selective perception, mind-reading, all or nothing thinking, emotive language, overgeneralisation)?

_____

_____

_____

_____

If you had an all-knowing, all-wise friend, how would s/he have seen the situation?

Is a reframing of the situation possible? (A glass that is half empty is also half full.)

What would your cost–benefit analysis be of seeing the situation the way you did?

_____

_____

_____

_____

A list of things you could do

Doing the right thing at the right time is one of the big secrets of conquering irritability. Some people are good at knowing what they want to do, but most of us benefit a lot from having a 'menu'. So here is such a menu, divided into headings just as a real menu would be. It is quite comprehensive, but you may wish to add things to it, cross some out, and 'adjust' others to suit you.

Entertainment

- Watch a movie on TV.
- Watch a documentary on TV.
- Watch a 'show' on TV.
- Watch a comedy.
- Listen to something informative on the radio.
- Listen to something light on the radio.
- Listen to some music.
- Choose a DVD to watch.
- Go to the cinema.
- Go to the theatre.
- Go to a club.
- Go to a sports event.
- Browse the Internet.
- Go on Facebook.
- Go on Twitter.
- Watch something on YouTube.
- Read a book/Kindle.
- Read a magazine.

- Read a newspaper.
- Play a game (cards, darts, board games).
- Do a hobby.
- Do some painting.
- Do some handicraft.
- Prepare a nice meal.

Exercise and biological

- Go for a walk.
- Do stretches.
- Go for a run.
- Go to the gym.
- Play football / basketball / baseball.
- Rowing, real or on machine.
- Have sex.
- Do some gardening.
- Wash the car.
- Have a short sleep.
- Practise dancing.

Do something for other people

- Help somebody with their gardening.
- Help somebody with their decorating.
- Do some shopping for somebody who needs it.
- Visit somebody who is in trouble or lonely.
- Do some organised charity work.
- Get in touch with somebody.

- Phone a friend.
- Phone a relative.
- Phone a work colleague or former work colleague.
- Phone a neighbour.
- Visit any of the above.
- Text or email any of the above.
- Write a letter to any of the above.
- Buy a present for somebody else.

Soothing activities

- Soak in the bath.
- Deliberately relax – do a relaxation exercise.
- Practise singing.
- Play the piano or other musical instrument.
- Eat a healthy meal.
- Walk around town.
- Go for a walk in the country.
- Write your diary.

Mental activities

- Plan my career or my future.
- Daydream my career or future.
- Daydream about good things from the past.
- Think about sex.
- Plan out tomorrow.
- Think about something you are looking forward to.
- Do a crossword or Sudoku.

- Study.
- Watch an educational programme.
- Read a newspaper.

Chores

(Note: these can also be enjoyable, at the right time!)
- Do some tidying.
- Do some cleaning.
- Get rid of old stuff.
- Repair something.
- Sort out the finances.
- Do some work.

Other

- Buy something from a shop.
- Buy something from the Internet.
- Rearrange some furniture.
- Go for a ride in the car, on the bike, or on a motorbike.

Useful Resources

ACT

Harris, R., *ACT Made Simple,* New Harbinger, 2009.

Hayes, S., Strosahl, K.D., and Wilson, K.G., *Acceptance and Commitment Therapy*, Guilford Press, 1999.

Anger and Aggression at Work

Davies, W. and Frude, N., *Preventing Face-to-face Violence: Dealing with Anger and Aggression at Work*, The APT Press, 1999.

Depression

Burns, D., *The Feeling Good Handbook*, Penguin, 1999.

Gilbert, P., *Overcoming Depression*, Robinson, 2009.

Gilbert, P., *Compassion Focused Therapy*, Taylor and Francis, 2010.

Diet

Davis, C.M., 'Results of the self-selection of diets by young children', *CMAJ (1939)*, 257–61 (available online).

Mindfulness

Kabat–Zin, J., *Mindfulness for Beginners: Reclaiming the Present Moment and Your Life,* Sounds True, *2012.*

Mood

Scott, J., *Overcoming Mood Swings*, Robinson, 2010.

Relationships

Crowe, M., *Overcoming Relationship Problems*, Robinson, 2005.

Sleep

Espie, C.A., *Overcoming Insomnia and Sleep Problems*, Robinson, 2006.

Stress

Brosan, L. and Todd, G., *Overcoming Stress*, Robinson, 2009.

McGonigal, K., *The Upside of Stress*, Avery, 2015.

Index

THE
IMPR⟳VEMENT
ZONE

Looking for life inspiration?

The Improvement Zone has it all, from **expert advice** on how to advance your **career** and boost your **business**, to improving your **relationships**, revitalising your **health** and developing your **mind**.

Whatever your goals, head to our website now.

www.improvementzone.co.uk

INSPIRATION ON THE MOVE

INSPIRATION DIRECT TO YOUR INBOX